BREAK YOUR LOVE AFFAIR WITH FOOD

How to Lose Weight Using the Law of Detachment

William F. McLaughlin

ISBN: 1490984550
ISBN-13: 9781490984551

THE LAW OF DETACHMENT:

Whatever you are attached to, controls and stresses you;

whatever you let go of, relaxes and frees you.

CONTENTS

INTRODUCTION

The Problem and the Remedy

The problem – and the premise of this book, is that the persistently overweight person *eats for emotional comfort instead of physical nourishment.* This wrong purpose and wrong relationship with food results in the virtual inability to control one's appetite, and is the root cause of overeating. Food temporarily helps the person feel comfortable and in control by alleviating negative emotions such as stress, boredom, worry, anger, loneliness, fear, etc.

This problem is corrected by learning to eat *without* emotional involvement. It's learning to eat *sensually* not emotionally. It's to separate or *detach* yourself from your feelings while you're eating. You want to eat *only* with the five senses – nothing else. You want to experience every moment, nuance and aspect of the eating process from an emotional *distance,* as if you're an outside observer or witness. You want to experience eating *objectively* as well as subjectively – experience it from the outside in as well as the inside out. The *Law of Detachment* is this: that to the degree you eat in this detached way, you recover natural control of your appetite, and your excess weight drops on its own.

Now this "Law of Detachment" is nothing new; it's as old as

humanity itself. It's the very "method" of being beautifully and powerfully free. It was taught by the greatest teachers in history. Take, for example, the saying of one of them, "Be in the world but not of the world." We could paraphrase it, "Be in your food but not of your food, " or "Be in your body but not of your body, " or "Eat to live; don't live to eat." And the essential teaching of another master was "The extinction of all attachment," – because, whatever you're attached to, controls you; whatever you're detached from, you control.

What *is* new, is that you'll be applying this universal law to achieve a specific, practical purpose – overcoming your Eating-for-Comfort Habit (ECH). You're going to cease being driven by any subconscious baggage from the past, however acquired. You'll learn to think, feel and eat, from a conscious *distance* instead of emotional attachment or entanglement. Living the Law of Detachment, then is the reality-based way to live a naturally healthy, happy, self-controlled life, a mind/body/spirit-controlled life. The purpose of this book is to show you how.

You'll learn what the law is and how to apply it to: *Recreating Your Self-Image, Controlling Your Appetite, Controlling Your Portions, Exercising Your Body, and Controlling Your Stress.*

CHAPTER 1

HOW TO RECREATE YOUR SELF-IMAGE

"The imagination is man's power over nature." – Wallace Stevens

The "Image-is-Reality" Principle

Overeating begins in the subconscious mind and spreads to the body, so the mind is where eighty percent of our work will be focused. The other twenty-percent is about diet and exercise.

Overeating, like any other habit, good or bad, is "programmed" into the subconscious, memory-bank part of your mind. This subconscious program *runs* your eating behavior automatically just as other programs run your respiratory and immune systems automatically.

Now this overeating habit can be controlled or changed at will, simply by saying the word, simply by telling it to do so. After all, you are the boss of your body – but you have to tell it in a certain way, a way that the subconscious part of your mind can understand and process.

How the Subconscious Mind Works

The first thing to understand about the subconscious mind is that it doesn't perceive or operate through eyes and ears, etc, because it doesn't have sense faculties. And it doesn't perceive or operate through thinking or feeling, because it doesn't have those faculties either. It can only perceive and operate according to the *image* that's presented or given to it. Let's say, for example, that you were taking a short-cut home through your neighbor's vegetable patch, and you bent over to tie your shoes – that would give the impression, perception, or image to anyone watching, that you were stealing a vegetable, wouldn't it? For the subconscious mind, the *image* of stealing is the *same* as actually stealing. It has the same effect. So for the subconscious mind, image *is* reality, perception *is* everything.

In other words, the subconscious mind sees and functions just like a computer program or mirror: If you give it "I can't do this," it will reflect "You can't do this"; If you give it "food makes me feel good," it will give you "food makes you feel good"; if you give it, "I am fat," it will give you "You are fat," – even if you're not. The essential point is this: If you look in the mirror and think or feel that there's something wrong with your body, or that you are overweight, then you're going to stay overweight for as long as you think that! So if you want to change how you look, feel and eat, you'll have to change your image accordingly. You'll have to imagine yourself *already* looking, feeling and eating the way you want. Your body follows your image like a train follows its tracks. This is what's meant by, "Be careful what you ask for," and, "It's all in your mind." That's because the subconscious mind is totally controlled by you, just as you are totally controlled by it. They mirror-reflect each other.

Your self-image is what's feeding and maintaining that body, so a new and improved self-image is how you're going to begin to change it. Your body will emulate your thinking whether your thinking is right or wrong, true or false. So if you're striving for a goal that contradicts what you "think" you presently are, then your subconscious must and will figure out a way to obstruct or sabotage your efforts. Your subconscious mirror reflects that you're overweight because that's what you put in front of it. Using the computer metaphor, your subconscious computer calculates that being overweight is what you want because that's the information you gave it.

This image-is-reality principle effects other areas of your life. For example, let's say you play Mahjong online, and for years you average a consistent fifty-three-percent rating. Then, without thinking at all about it, you're rating improves to sixty-five percent – much better than your subconscious is programmed to "think" is your rating. So you proceed to subconsciously sabotage subsequent matches by, for example, matching wrong pairs, and finding yourself stuck with unmatchable tiles blocking other key tiles, so you can't clear the layout, etc., – all to bring you back to the fifty-three percent rating you've accepted as yours – back to your secure "comfort zone" of everything being just as it has always been.

Changing Your Self-Image

You change your self-image by *convincing* the subconscious mind that you're *not* overweight. It will then slap immediate controls on your appetite to make this imaginary fact a real fact.

In changing your self-image, there are several elements to understand and follow. The first element is to mentally change from the weight (or eating behavior) you presently are to that which you desire to be. We'll refer to that as your "default" weight. You want to see and feel yourself as your ideal weight right *here and now*, even though your "logical" mind tells you that you're really not. This is because when it comes to any eating disorder, it doesn't matter what your logical mind thinks. *Your logical mind didn't get you overweight and your logical mind won't get you thinner* – as you may have noticed. You can't use the same mind that caused the problem to correct it. That's why you have to use your imagination instead of logic. Logic is doing what you've always done – like dieting, because that's how you've always done it. It doesn't work because "if nothing changes, nothing changes." Your vivid imagination has the power to override or transcend logic to bring your goal to realization. So it's not about changing your diet program; it's about changing your subconscious-mind program.

Resetting Your Default Weight

Someone said, "I always wanted to be somebody, but I should've been more specific." That's a humorous observation – and it's true because the subconscious mind requires that your goal be specific. Only when the goal is clearly defined, can the subconscious begin to process your order. Specificity is a necessary factor in convincing your subconscious that you've *already* arrived, that that's who you "really" are right here and now. Just as you can't feed approximate numbers into your home computer, so you can't to your subconscious computer.

Let's say you determine your ideal weight to be exactly 135 pounds, and your present weight is 178 pounds. That means you want to lose exactly 43 pounds. The next step is to determine exactly how many pounds per week you want to lose, and that'll give your exact goal date. All the numbers you choose here should to be wise and feasible. They have to be "okay" with your subconscious, based on past performance. This means that if you're at all uncomfortable or uncertain about a number, it may be counterproductive. Your subconscious may "balk" at it. Also remember that you're just in the planning stage now, just initiating the creative process. All these numbers can be modified or even discarded after they've been internalized.

Let's say you choose to lose exactly three pounds per week. Dividing 43 by 3, you get a target date of 14 1/3 weeks. That's 14 weeks, 2 days, and 8 hours. Yes, count the hours too.

What has this to do with detachment? By virtue of following an exact plan, with exact numbers you, in effect, *remove* your old self, your old self-image, from the decision-making process. And to remove yourself is to detach yourself.

What you're doing is putting yourself on automatic pilot – which is how you've been operating in the past; the difference now is that you're *not* on overeating-autopilot, you're on losing-weight-autopilot. You're eating now from the dictates of free-will, instead of compulsion.

Internalizing Your Goal

The question now is how to instill your goal weight or behavior into the subconscious so it becomes natural and second nature to you. This is done by simply affirming it to yourself, but you have to affirm it in a certain way, otherwise it'll just go in one ear and out the other. It has to reach deep into the subconscious mind, the source and instrument of mind/body change. In other words, for the affirmation to work, it has to *sink in.* It has to be assimilated or *internalized*. Remember that the purpose of the affirmation is to *convince* the subconscious that your goal weight or behavior is your *current* weight or behavior. This could take hours, days or even weeks, depending how averse to change is the security-blanket part of your mind.

The internalization experience is similar to that of losing a loved one, especially when the loss is sudden or unexpected. The loss doesn't "hit" you for some time afterward. It took time for your loss to sink in and be accepted as true. Only then does the mourning process begin. In the same way, the appetite-control process can't begin until your goal weight has sunk in. Your goal has to as if percolate through the hindering, logical part of your mind, the part that inexplicably fears change. Think of the logical mind as a security guard on constant alert. It wants to "protect" you from entering the door to the scary, subconscious unknown. But its error is – that's exactly the door to your appetite-control power.

Just repeat the statement, to yourself or softly aloud, "I am (135) pounds!" The most powerful prefix to use in any mantra or affirmation are the words "I am," because no other words, according to eastern meditation masters, initiate the creative process more effectively. No other words go so directly to the heart or seat of power. Repeat the affirmation many times throughout the day, especially at mealtimes. The best times are when you're in that relaxed, drowsy state when just waking in the morning and at bedtime when you're just on the verge of sleep. That's when your robotic security guard is most down. Repeat it for several minutes. Your intuition will tell you when the words are starting to sink in or becoming more meaningful. You can create or deepen that relaxed state at any time by using some kind of relaxation or meditation exercise – one of which is described in Chapter 7.

Relaxing Your Guard

The way to neutralize that entrenched, eating-for-comfort security guard is simply to *relax* her. Relax her to the point her guard is down enough to allow your new weight or eating behavior to be accepted into your creative subconscious mind. That's the germination point where the blooming of the new you can begin.

The way to access the subconscious part of your mind is by relaxing the conscious part. The conscious part is almost always moving – constantly thinking, reasoning, desiring, analyzing, rationalizing, conceptualizing – while the subconscious part is constantly *still*. The idea is to still the conscious mind to the same level as is the subconscious mind. That's the point of exchange when your goal affirmation can transfer to it. The process is like that of an airplane being refueled in midair by another airplane. The transfer of fuel can only take place when both planes are moving at the same speed at the same time. Or think of the opening of the subconscious mind as the eye of a relaxed sewing needle, and the conscious mind as a nervous length of thread. The thread must be stilled before it can pass through the eye of the needle.

The relationship between the conscious and subconscious mind is a communication process much like that between a radio receiver and transmitter. The transmitter is like the subconscious mind. It is the *source* of all intelligence and goal-achievement power. And the receiver is like the conscious mind. Its job is to be *receptive* to the source. It can't be receptive, however, unless it's tuned into the transmitter, and it can't unless it (the dial) is still or relaxed.

When we are excited or stressed, it's as if we are chaotically and indiscriminately moving the dial hither and dither, back and forth, without ever coming to rest, and so receiving only gibberish as a result. We're scattered rather than focused.

Or think of the conscious and subconscious minds as the two sections of an hourglass: The subconscious is the top half, and only about seven-percent at a time can ever flow into consciousness, the bottom half. The narrow-minded (biased) neck restricts the flow. As we become more open-minded through detachment, we in effect, widen the neck of the hourglass until it becomes like a water glass. Now, what's above is the same as below. Now there's no difference between the top-half and the bottom-half. Now they are one whole, not two halves. One mind, not two minds. There's no separation, obstruction, conflict or distinction between them. What was subconscious now becomes conscious. At that point, you are empowered! Whatever state of body or mind you want is yours, first imaginatively, then in due course, physically. You realize natural and effortless appetite-control power, and the excess weight drops of its own accord. Or in the case of other eating disorders, the behavior falls away on its own. It just gives up on you because you're no longer feeding or empowering it.

The "Happiness-First" Principle

We can now move on to the next element in the mind/body transformation process. Earlier I defined an "eating disorder" as the condition when the mind follows the body instead of vice versa. This means that you have to change your mind before the body can change. So we're not talking at all about "dieting" here; that's putting the body first instead of the mind first, which is the erroneous, upside-down approach guaranteed to fail every time. The correct approach is to begin at the *end* not the beginning. By the "end" we not only mean your goal weight, we also and especially mean *the state of mind to which your goal will bring you* – and that is a state of *happiness,* isn't it?

Yes, achieving your goal will make you happy, but the catch – the paradoxical law governing the creative process is that *you must be happy before you can control your appetite and lose that weight.* Happiness is the seed; weight loss is the fruit. You have to be happy in the first place before you can lose weight in the second place. Happy in, happy out. What goes around, comes around. What gives, gets.

So what is the definition of happiness in this context? Happiness is a state of *perfect contentment* in which there are no needs or desires. It is a state of equilibrium or centeredness – which is the highest state of mind to which one can aspire because, in a world of opposites, conflicts and contradictions, there is simply nothing higher than *centered.* It is a state of mind so peaceful, harmonious and joyful, that all the rest of life is worthless in comparison. It is the very meaning and purpose of life; the whole aim and end of human existence. It means you've arrived.

But many of us have been ineffective in realizing true happiness and the goal-achieving power that comes with it. The reason is twofold: first, we are chasing what we already possess – which the masters have been trying to teach us throughout history. True happiness, as opposed to emotional happiness, is our case right now. It's not a thing to be sought externally, but is an inherent potential to be realized from within. It's not something apart from or alien to us. It is our first name, our very nature and constitution. It is always just at hand. To chase something we already possess is like a dog chasing its own tail. The more he pursues it emotionally, the more it eludes him and the more frustrated he becomes. We are in a state of happiness right now but don't realize it, just as the dog already has his tail but doesn't realize it.

Some smart dogs, however, do realize they are chasing their own tails but do it just for the fun of it. For them, catching their tails is not the object of the game: *the object is the chase itself.* This is the second thing we're doing wrong – making the object more important than the chase. Happiness lies in the *impersonal pursuit* of an object or ideal, not the *conquest* of it. The conquest is a mere formality, for when the object is caught it means the end of the game. And we don't want the game to ever end because that's the whole beauty and joy of life. A cat, for example, lives only to catch a mouse. That's his whole reason for being. It's how he's designed. He spends many of his waking hours preparing and practicing to catch a mouse – even though he may have never seen one. But when he finally does catch one – it's anticlimactic. He quickly becomes bored and will try to prolong the chase by poking and prodding the mouse into fleeing again. But the mouse soon dies and the cat is left despondent knowing that the game is over. When the mouse died, the cat effectively died too.

This principle that true happiness, as opposed to emotional happiness, lies in creative pursuit rather than in the conquest can be similarly observed when we lose an adversary or a loved one: When an adversary dies, we don't necessarily feel relief as might be expected, but rather a sense of loss. We had been at odds for so long, that our resentment had become habitual. We carried it around with us. We came to enjoy resenting that person. It gave us a life. We got some morbid pleasure out of it. So when he leaves or dies, we're not glad but feel an emptiness much like the cat whose mouse had died. We don't really miss the *person,* we miss the resenting (the pursuing), for if we have anger within us, one person is as good as another. The object of our resentment is secondary; the primary thing is the ongoing activity of resenting. And likewise when we lose a loved one, we don't really grieve the loss of the *person* himself but the loss of the *loving* of that person. The *object* of our love is secondary to the loving itself, for if we have love within us, one person is as good as another. It's the loving itself that we relish, not the person; the person is just a medium.

True happiness, then, isn't found *in* people, places and things, but *through* them. Our work and relationships are the field, medium or means through which the happiness within may be realized and expressed. Similarly, happiness is realized *through* listening to good music, watching a colorful sunset, tasting a delicious apple, feeding a sparrow, smelling a rose, building a better can opener. Music is not important, but listening is; food is not the thing, taste and nourishment are; flowers are not important; their beauty and fragrance are. A better can opener is not the essential thing; being creative is. These "activities" serve to draw out the spirit of happiness latent within us. They act as spurs or catalyzing devices. A flower means nothing in and of itself; it is only when the color, form and fragrance of it agree, harmonizes or relates to complementary qualities within us that we experience beauty and joy. This is how we become one with the flower.

The essence of all this is that happiness isn't something that happens by accident, but is a moment-to-moment, conscious, recreational activity. To create something means to discover or draw out that which *already* exists on some level. Happiness already exists to an infinite degree. All that remains is to realize it more and more, to uncover it more and more. Life itself has no purpose that needs to be fulfilled. It has *already* been purposed and fully filled. It is done. Life has nothing else to do but be discovered, and we have nothing else to do but discover it. Life has nothing else to do but give and we, to partake. Life is ever the lover and we are ever the beloved.

Life is a game or recreational activity whose object is to continually discover this inner happiness, this "most high" thing within us and then to share it with others. Everything else is secondary, superficial and subordinate. You can call it finding freedom, finding your higher self, finding God, Truth, Love,

Christ, nirvana, enlightenment, heaven, reality. It doesn't matter what word or symbol you use. What matters is what it *is*, what it means. The meaning of life is to realize it has no universal meaning; it has only a *personal* meaning. It's whatever you personally say it is from moment to moment. It is you who give life and everything in it its meaning. Life, consciousness and happiness are all there is and all there has to be. It is only when we're *not* alive, aware or happy that we futilely attempt to invent false purpose and meaning.

What, then, is personally meaningful to you in your life right now? What goal do you have that will recreate or trigger your innate happiness? What is it that you desire? Desire is the door opener, the impetus, the stimulus. What is it that will "make" you happy and content at this particular time and place in your life? You say you want to lose that excess weight you've been carrying around for so long. You want to regain control of your body, control of your appetite, control of your health, happiness and appearance. In other words, you want *power* over your life.

How to Desire

The paradoxical problem in achieving your goal is that emotional desire is almost always accompanied with stress or anxiety. They come as a package – two sides of the same coin. Desire contradicts contentment. Desire indicates something is missing. There is a lack or deficiency. Whenever you feel in want or need of something, you leave the realm of relaxed and joyful contentedness and become tense like a tightly stretched rubber band. You become off-center, unbalanced, and you remain so until that goal is fulfilled, satisfied or resolved in some way. The *emotional* effort to achieve that goal is what strengthens the disorder's grip on you – it's exactly what hinders recovery.

We are almost always stressed because we are almost always wanting something or other. The human being is a virtual *desiring machine.* We want to grow, improve, evolve, expand. We want more money, more security, more sex, more time, more space, more power. We want to improve our bridge game, have a better car, a better job, a better relationship, a bigger house, a faster computer. We want to get married or divorced, buy a boat or get rid of a boat, get justice or revenge, pass that test, improve our health, heal a disease, make a good impression, be right, be first, be famous, be more attractive, wiser and wittier; be more recognized, validated, admired, appreciated. We want to win the race, win the argument, get that promotion, retire early. The list is seemingly endless and constant.

The conundrum is this: You're stressed *because* you emotionally want something, and that clarity-blocking stress is exactly what prevents you from getting it. It's a vicious cycle. So the essential question becomes – how can you *desire* to lose weight, for example, without the failure-causing stress that comes with it? In other words, how can you be happy *before* you lose that weight, so that you *can* lose that weight?

The Principle of "Already-Being-There"

The answer lies in knowing *the right way to desire.* It's about knowing the "lawful" way to ask yourself for the weight or behavior that you want. Now, your computer-like subconscious requires certain criteria be met before it can process your order. The first is that you order with the right attitude, and the right attitude is to assume, believe and accept that you *already* have, right now, whatever you desire to be, do or have. Again, you have to be there in mind before you can be there in body – as we discussed earlier. You have to mentally and emotionally accept as a foregone conclusion, as a *fait accompli*, that your goal has *already* been achieved, that it's a done deal, that it's finished.

This attitude of "already being there" overrides or transcends the desire-stress-failure vicious cycle. You are now like a plane flying above the storm. You are now, in effect, not only happily content in the *process* of losing that weight, you are now most effective in losing it. Emotional-control *is* appetite-control. They are one and the same state of mind. You are unstoppable because you're living above and detached from all that could or would block you. Assuming that you've "already arrived" empowers your subconscious to make it happen in reality by removing failure-causing emotionality from the goal-achievement process.

You are formulating your desire in a way that conforms with how the imaginative, creative faculty is designed to work, with how the subconscious mind is actually wired. You are in compliance with subconscious law.

Now everything in the universe works according to law and order, and the mind is no exception. The law of your mind, that is, your higher, subconscious mind, is that it *must* give you whatever you want or need. You are the law of yourself, the boss of yourself, the boss of your body. Think of the subconscious as your personal computer and you are its master programmer. Whatever you say, goes. You just have to say it in the right way – beginning with the attitude you *already* have it.

Here's a variation of an old Zen story that illustrates the above point: An American woman, despairingly overweight for many years, traveled to the Himalayas to seek the counsel of a famous wise woman. After much searching, she found her walking up a steep hill. The American struggled to catch up to her.

The wise woman said, "Why do you want to see me?"

The American said, "Please, I want to lose weight. I want to lose weight."

"The way to lose weight," said the wise woman, "can be stated in five words."

"Five words? But, I've traveled such a long way," said the American. "Can you give me more than just five words?"

"I can give you ten-thousand words if you like, but they would boil down to the same five words."

"Okay," said the American. "I've tried everything. Tell me what to do and I will do it. What are the five words?"

"Just drop the '*I want*,'" said the wise woman.

You overcome the vicious circle by getting out of the way of it. You put your lower, personal, emotional self aside, in order to fulfill the law and achieve your goal. You have to separate yourself from what you want in order for your higher, subconscious self, to proceed to give it to you. Detachment, again and again, is the master key to the emotional-control that *is* appetite-control. It's removing yourself from, or rising above, the emotional desire to lose that weight by assuming and accepting that you've already lost it.

You are coming from success not from hunger or deficiency. Deficient is not who you are. That's a deception. You are whole and complete, just as the universe is. So all your desires and goals are merely recreational activities that can't fail to be achieved because on some level, they already are. That's the reality-based way to think of them.

You are now, in effect, emotionally uninvolved regarding the end result. It's not a factor in the success equation. You are totally indifferent and dispassionate with respect to the whether or not you lose that weight or reverse that disorder. This is how you facilitate the achievement process rather than short-circuit or sabotage it. Henry James put it this way – "When once a decision is reached and execution is the order of the day, dismiss absolutely all responsibility and care about the outcome."

Extricating (detaching) yourself emotionally from your goal is the means by which to access the joy, clarity and creative power necessary to achieve that goal. The inspiration of the painter, poet, composer, entrepreneur, etc., comes only when he's able to view his work with emotional detachment. He becomes tense when ideas don't flow, and when they do, excitement prevents their sustainment. He suffers frustration because what he clearly knows in his mind and feels in his heart won't translate faithfully onto a canvas or into words or music. He's blocked. Uncontrolled emotion has stifled his power of perception and expression.

The creative genius in any medium is one who has learned to overcome a restless mind and an anxious heart. He can maintain a serene indifference during both the creative feasts and famines alike; consequently, the famines occur less and less, and the feasts, more and more. The same principle of creative success applies to the appetite-control artist. Non-emotional involvement with food is the master key to achieving control over it.

Failure is not a factor; not a consideration. It is unthinkable. A virtual impossibility. It does not even enter the realm of imagination. So-called failure is nothing but positive feedback, to inform you that you slipped off center, off the right attitude. You've slipped back to emotional attachment. It is not something to give up over. This is why giving up is never, ever an option. Failure is always just a misunderstanding. It's like the classic Greek tragedy of a man who committed suicide because he thought his beloved committed suicide; but she committed suicide because she mistakenly thought he had.

Just let the subconscious do all the work. Keep your lower, personal, hungry self out of the picture. Your best thinking got you into this situation; don't depend on it to get you out of it. Only when you are above and detached from your feelings can your feelings be controlled and your desire be granted. It is granted first on the subconscious level the moment you ask in this way, then, in due course, it's granted in actuality – on the physical level. In other words, you control your emotions in order to control the outcome, and you control your emotions by keeping a *distance* from them.

To assume you're "already there" entails *visualizing what you'll look and feel like at your goal weight.* Creative imagination is the forming of a picture in the mind's eye of what you want to be, do or have. In cinematic terms, you'd be creating a "trailer" of your future body, or a "preview of coming attractions." Or we could say, "A preview of coming attractiveness." Imagining a thing is prerequisite to having it in actuality. This is creative law, and it applies to creating the mind and body that you want, just as to creating the house, business, relationships, etc. that you want.

The Right Motivation

Let's clarify a few foundational points before you begin to visualize your present-future body. First, the creative process requires that you desire to achieve your goal for the right reason or right motivation. The right motivation gives you the necessary resoluteness and firmness of purpose to overwrite the long-established false program that keeps you in the grip of your eating disorder. Think of your subconscious mind as the negative in a camera. In order to impress upon it the *picture* of the mind and body that you want, the light of your desire has to be sufficiently intense.

Natural and lasting appetite-control has to be your heart's burning, dominant desire. You have to be irrevocably and unwaveringly determined as well as happily detached and centered. Gaining control of your mind and body has to be the number-one priority in your life, not only for itself, but also because it affects every other area of your life. Along with your appearance and health, it affects your self-confidence, self-esteem and self-image. It affects your relationships, your finances, your work and your play.

You can't achieve your goal for your spouse, children, boyfriend – or even for your job, health or appearance. You can't lose weight for that Caribbean cruise, or the upcoming wedding of your daughter, or to get into that undersized designer suit you bought on sale, etc. The only motivation the subconscious mind can respond to is one that is primal, as primal as survival itself. It must come from the source or center of your being – and that right motivation is *total self-control, power and freedom!* That's what you *really* want if you go deeply enough into the question. No one wants to live with a "monkey on his back," or an "elephant in the room." No one wants to be a junkie or an addict. No one wants any area of her life out of control. No one wants to feel insecure or powerless in any way. Self-controlled freedom is the only motivation that will work because free-will is our strongest, most essential human need and desire, our most precious birthright.

Willpower Versus Perseverance

Many people on the path of recovery from their food issues often cite a lack of sufficient willpower as the main reason for their setbacks. But they have plenty of willpower or they wouldn't have tried so many remedies so many times. The problem is they just don't know how to use willpower. The incorrect understanding and use of willpower is the most common reason for failure in any long-term endeavor

Willpower isn't designed for long-term use – such as running a marathon or maintaining lifelong self-control. It's designed only for short bursts of energy and adrenalin – like being able to lift a two-thousand pound car to save a child's life, for instance – but you wouldn't be able to hold it up for very long, would you?

Instead of using willpower to achieve your goal, use *patient perseverance*. Willpower and perseverance seem alike, but are different faculties with different purposes. Willpower is a lower mental faculty, while perseverance or determination is a faculty of the heart or center. Willpower is a state of doing, while perseverance is a state of being. Perseverance doesn't use any energy at all so can be "practiced" constantly and indefinitely. Mental willpower, on the other hand, is limited and quickly spent.

You may have noticed that whenever you've tried willpower to lose weight, for example, you burned out quickly. You became drained, began to lose confidence and doubt yourself. Each time you attempt willpower to control yourself, you'll fail, and you'll fail sooner each time, because you just know that you're going to fail – and of course, you will because you're using the wrong tool in the wrong way.

So instead of using willpower to achieve your goal, use patient perseverance – which is just cool, calm, old-fashioned stick-to-it-iveness. You just *know* you're on the right track and just *know* you're going to get there. Patient perseverance is the opposite of "willfulness." Willfulness is a self-centered, egotistical pushing, while perseverance is a centered, detached, positive movement. One works, the other doesn't. One backfires, the other propels you unstoppably toward your goal.

The next question is, to what are you going to apply this patient perseverance? You're going to apply it to recreating your self-image – which is a creative process. It's creative in that it utilizes the *imagination* – as any goal-oriented activity does – like writing a novel or running a business. If you want to build something you have to visualize it first, plan it out in your mind first, don't you? You're going to use your imagination to visualize yourself at your desired weight, and feeling very happy about it.

This creative visualization process is essential because *mind/body change is predicated upon self-image.* It's determined by it. Your new self-image will be the essential foundation and model for your mind/body transformation.

Creating Yourself in Your Own Image

As your mind is a desiring machine, it's also a creating machine. You couldn't have that desire to lose weight within you unless you also had the means of fulfillment already within you as well. They are two sides of the same mind. In order for your subconscious to fulfill your desire, it needs a clear *picture* of the finished product. It has to see with complete clarity and certitude exactly what it's supposed to create. For the subconscious mind, seeing is believing and accepting. If you can picture it, you virtually have it. The rest is just process, just follow-up. Before you can *physically* produce that better mouse trap you have in mind, you have to put on paper a minutely-detailed diagram of it. The more detailed the better. In other words, you will need a model or archetype to emulate and replicate.

This is where your imagination comes into play. You want to draw a vivid mental picture of your proposed body and keep it in the forefront of your mind. Memorize it. You want to stamp this image onto your subconscious memory bank – superimpose it over the current image of yourself. Incorporate it – as we talked about earlier. This is how a "method" actor gets into his role. He becomes his role by convincing/imagining that he really is the character he's going to play. Then when the director says "action,"the actor plays the character perfectly because he programmed his subconscious mind that that's who he is.

All the great athletes do the same. They first visualize making the perfect movement, shot or swing, then perform exactly how they pre-imagined they would. The great golfer's ball doesn't land in bunkers or traps because in the visualization of the swing, they don't exist.

The subconscious mind can't discriminate between what's real and what's vividly imagined. For example, if you were walking along a path in a park, and a branch fell from a tree and you thought it was a snake – you'd react as if it were a snake. Your heart rate would increase. Adrenalin would start pumping. Cortisol levels would rise. Muscles would tense. You'd start sweating and hyperventilating, etc. – but it's merely a piece of wood! This is similar to the "placebo effect" whereby if you *believe* a particular pill will cure your illness, it will have an amazing tendency to cure that illness even though that pill may contain nothing but sugar.

In the same way, you want the subconscious to *believe* that you already have the body you want. It will then proceed to affect all systems to coincide with that vision. It will affect the serotonin, endorphin, cortisol, metabolic and hormonal levels and speeds, etc. to facilitate the creation of that body. Along with the appropriate physiological changes, it will also inform your conscious mind when you've eaten the correct amount of food. It will bring about satiety on lesser amounts of food than usual. It will make you more discriminating as to the quality, freshness and naturalness of food. It will make junk food unappealing. It will diminish between-meal craving. It will facilitate digestion, etc. The output of the subconscious mind will perfectly reproduce the input to the degree the input is specific and the image is vivid. Just as overeating began in the mind and spread to the body, so the correction begins in the mind and spreads to the body.

Believe Yourself Recovered

Countless volumes have been written on the power of faith, and all of the greatest teachers of self-mastery throughout history have proved and taught the efficacy of faith. No matter how clear and strong your desire to lose that weight, if you don't *believe* that you can and will do it, then you can't and won't. It's simple mathematics. Henry Ford said, "Whether you *do* believe you can do it or *don't* believe you can do it – you're right." He knew that success or failure is not only a state of mind, it's also a *choice* of mind. You can choose to believe you can control your appetite, or not. You want to doubt your doubts more and believe your beliefs more.

The subconscious computer doesn't care or lean one way or the other. The subconscious mind is your free-will faculty – totally impersonal and indifferent. Whatever you tell it, it will accept. Whatever you ask of it in the right way, it *must* give you because that's its job, its primary purpose. Any fear, doubt or uncertainty about attaining this goal is asking incorrectly. It's asking with attachment to the goal. It's asking in a contradictory way – as if you don't already have it, and that's exactly what will prevent success. What else can be expected? The process has been sabotaged at its inception, before it can even begin. Disappointment is a forgone conclusion. Doubt, worry or uncertainty is virtually planning to fail, and so you will.

The subconscious mind will accept your goal mind and body exactly as presented, exactly as imagined, whether it's right or wrong, true or false, healthy or unhealthy. It isn't at all logical like the conscious mind. It doesn't discriminate, analyze, rationalize or judge. If you ask for something in the right way – the detached, desireless way prescribed here, it will be granted. Period. It is the law of cause and effect.

So faith is really more scientific than commonly understood. It's just as exact a science as mathematics. Just because you can't see the future doesn't mean it doesn't exist. And not only does it exist, but you can create it or re-create it the way you want it. If you can imagine it, you can have it. And nothing can stop you except your own disbelief.

Any fear, doubt or uncertainty about losing that weight or recovering from any other eating disorder are your own mental concoctions and have no basis in objective reality. All such negative thoughts are self-created concepts based mostly on perceived failures and baggage from the past. If you come from past mistakes or so-called failures, you are bound to repeat them. In reality, nothing more can be expected. If you come from the clear, unencumbered, open-minded present, your future mind/body is yours for the defining and asking.

The "Self-Esteem-First" Principle

Reality is whatever you think or imagine it is, so think of this new body as the real you – as real and present as the air you breathe; while your past body is not real in the sense that it doesn't express or fulfill the real you. Now just because that old body is not really you doesn't mean you should dislike it. If you dislike your body or hold yourself in low esteem because of it, you will *never* control your appetite and lose that weight – because you're living under a false premise. Your old mind/body is not at fault. Your old mind/body is the *effect* of something not the cause of something. Your old mind/body is totally innocent.

This is why unconditional love of your current self and body is prerequisite to achieving your goal just as happiness-first is prerequisite. Acceptance allows and empowers change while fat-like rejection sticks to you like a magnet. Accepting your body and yourself just as they are is the first element on the ladder of change. This is called living life on life's terms. It's living in reality. You can't change the universe but you can change your attitude and response to it. You can't control the wind, but you can adjust the sails.

Love yourself with all your heart, soul, mind and strength, and never doubt yourself for an instant. Again, doubt all your doubts. There are no accidents in the universe. You had to go through all you went through in order to come to this final stage of freedom and recovery. The Buddha said, "You can search throughout the entire universe for someone who is more deserving of your love and affection than you are yourself, and that person is not to be found anywhere. You yourself, as much as anybody in the entire universe deserve your love and affection."

Instead of doubting success, just be open to it. Be amenable to it. Self-control is not something you do; it's something you *allow*. When you doubt or fear, you are effectively separating yourself from your goal. You are putting your ideal body on an emotional pedestal, programming yourself to remain always apart from it. Doubt puts your goal over the horizon somewhere where it must always remain. When you doubt, you are like *Waiting for Godot*. Godot will never come. Waiting, trying, and doubting then become a way of life, just as running from diet to diet becomes a way of life. Doubting makes your goal an unattainable object, an ongoing exercise in futility and fantasy like a carrot held in front of one's nose. Either control your appetite or don't control it, but don't doubt and don't try. Just do it! The subconscious only understands do or die. It's a binary thing. Yes or no. Have or have not. It can't compute the indecisiveness, uncertainty and weakness of doubt, fear, hope, try or maybe. So doubt all your doubts and believe all your beliefs.

To be open-minded and acceptant is to be empty and receptive. Whenever you're empty, all that's necessary to achieve your goal will effortlessly rush in to fill the void. Emerson said, "Once you make a decision, the universe conspires to make it happen." If you want something, you have to make a space for it. That's what detachment does and that's what it means.

Mirror, Mirror, On the Wall

Several times daily, practice picturing yourself at your goal weight or condition. If this is difficult for you, then use a photograph of you when you were the size you want to return to. Or use a photo of a celebrity whose body you can use as a guideline. If you have photo-editing software on your computer, place your head on that body. If not, just cut and paste your head onto the body. Put copies on your refrigerator, closet and all your mirrors.

You're changing your mind and that new mind is now changing your body, and you fully allow and accept this change. You accept this new self-image as the true you. You accept that you've moved onto a higher and leaner plane of existence and consciousness. You're no longer stuck in that emotion-driven body, no longer stuck in that false image of yourself.

You now see yourself as a lean person sees herself. You conduct yourself as a lean person conducts herself. You live as a lean person lives. You think and feel as a lean person thinks and feels. You act and speak as a lean person acts and speaks. You eat as a lean person eats. You face life as lean person faces life.

Now use your best imagination to see yourself, as if from distance, as if witnessing yourself on a large movie screen. You're standing in front of a full-length wall mirror. You step onto your bathroom scale and see it point to your current weight of (178) pounds. Now look up and see your current body in the mirror. You don't judge your body in any way; just look at it impersonally, indifferently. You don't see it as *your* body any longer, as you've achieved some degree of detachment already. You just see it as just a body. You begin to realize that this is not your real body in a sense, not the real you, not an *expression* of the real you. You look at your hair and see that your hair is an expression of you. You glance over at the clothes in your closet and know that all those clothes are expressions of you. You look around and see that the contents of your home and your home itself, and the car in your driveway are direct reflections of you.

You realize that your whole life – your friends, work, hobbies, books, etc., are perfect reflections of your personality. But what of this excess weight? This isn't you. You are not at all resentful about it, but it simply isn't you. This excess weight does not express you. It's not part of your present makeup or mindset at all. It has nothing to do with who and what you really are. It's an aberration. So you let it go. You don't have to go to a psychiatrist for ten years. The problem is *now* and is dropped *now*. Whatever happened in your past is now irrelevant. In a single swoop, you drop the past with all its conscious or unconscious programming and conditioning. Everything in your life that has ever caused or has anything whatsoever to do with this excess weight, you let it go. You drop it like a hot, fat potato. You have the power and the tools now to do it and be it. And nothing can stop you. No person, place or thing can stop you.

You relax now. Your mind becomes quiet and still as you detachedly focus on this body in the mirror. You have a very powerful imagination. Imagine yourself at your perfect size and shape. Run your magic hands over your body and shape it into the form you desire. A student of Rodin asked him to explain, in the simplest terms, how to sculpt – an elephant, for example. Rodin said, "That is easy. Just take a chunk of marble, and with your hammer and chisel remove everything from it that is *not* an elephant." That's what you want to do.

Using your imagination as hammer and chisel, remove any extraneous fat from your body, all the fat that is not the real you. Notice that the excess fat and cellulite are loosening and dissolving – especially on those parts of the body that you want the fat off. You feel yourself becoming lighter and lighter. Look down at the scale and see the pointer gradually, almost imperceptively, moving to a lower and lower number until it finally stops exactly on your goal weight. You are neither surprised nor amazed, but calmly accept your new body as your real body. This is the new way it is. You wonder where you've been all these years.

When you have a clear picture of you at your desired weight, walk slowly toward that attractive image in the mirror, all the way up to that image – then step into that mirror – like *Alice in Wonderland*, and become one with that image.

Now see yourself getting dressed, putting on that great black suit you haven't been able to get into in years – the one you've been saving for this moment. You feel the smooth, soft material against your skin. The smell of that old wool is delightful. Now see your new self shopping at the mall and notice heads turning to have a second look at you. See yourself at work – clothes hanging loose and comfortable. See yourself exercising at the gym – and loving it. See yourself at a social event laughing with friends, etc.

Feeling Now The Way You Will Feel Then

Vividly picturing yourself at your goal weight is only one of the two components necessary to transformation – the physical part. The other part is *emotional*. Your emotional response needs to be *now* what it'll be when you've actually arrived at your target weight or behavior – which is happy! You have to add to that picture the feeling of joy, contentment, pride, satisfaction and fulfillment that you'll feel when that body is realized or actualized on your target date. This is part of both, the Self-Esteem-First and the Happiness-First principles we discussed earlier. You want to fill that picture with light and love. You feel good about your life now. You feel finally in control of it now. You feel free now and this makes you extremely happy.

To help conjure up that feeling of joy and contentment, use another technique of the "method" actor. Look back over your life to a time or situation when you remember feeling immense happiness. Perhaps, for example, when you rode your first bicycle, or when you graduated high school or college, or fell in love, or got married, had a child, got a promotion, or hit the lottery, etc. Then every time you envision your goal body, affix to it that joyful memory. Emotionalize that image. Replay this happy picture constantly through the day. Practice being happy all the time no matter what, because that's what you really are. Practice will bring you to realize it.

Let's close chapter 1 noting the key points and principles to remember:

1. That, overeating is a *subconscious habit* where the body controls the mind instead of mind controlling the body (mind over matter);

2. That mind/body change is predicated on *self-image*, not logic or intellect;

3. That you begin to change your self-image by *convincing* the subconscious mind, via affirmation, that you've *already* reached your goal weight or behavior;

4. That you have to be happy and content *before* you can achieve your goal;

5. That to prevent the goal-blocking stress of emotional desire, you proceed toward your goal with the firm conviction that you've *already* achieved it;

6. That your primary motivation for achieving your goal must be *freedom and self-control* – power over your life;

7. That you proceed toward your goal utilizing *patient perseverance* instead of mental willpower;

8. That the law of your subconscious mind *must* give you what you want; so believe without a shadow of doubt, fear or uncertainty that your goal is achieved;

9. That you must love and respect yourself and your body *before* you can achieve your goal;

10. That you have to *vividly picture and happily feel* yourself at your goal weight or behavior. Take it for granted – but with gratitude and humility, that you're already there.

Holding that super-clear, joyful image as a creative foundation, you can now begin transforming it into physical reality.

CHAPTER 2

HOW TO CONTROL YOUR APPETITE

"Every battle is won before it's ever fought." – SunTzu

How the Love Affair Began

Understanding the root cause of overeating is necessary in order to recover from it. Ignorance isn't bliss; it's fattening. You don't want merely temporary, symptomatic relief. You know from painful and expensive trial and error, through diet after diet, that doesn't work. You want lasting, causal, reality-based relief. You want a natural way of being and eating you can live with, one you can "practice" for life.

How did this eating problem arise? Why and how did you gain that excess weight in the first place? Why is it so hard to get rid of? And how can you get rid of it steadily, naturally, and without stress, strain or deprivation? In other words, you want to know what makes you tick. Socrates said, "Know thyself." When you know yourself, you know virtually everything, including how to regain control of your appetite and lose that weight once and for all.

All self-satisfying excuses, reasons, rationalizations and justifications aside, you're overweight because you overeat, and you overeat because you eat for the wrong reason: *You eat for emotional security or comfort instead of for physical nourishment.* You eat to *feel* good, and anything that makes you feel good you want more and more of it. You hate to stop eating because as soon as you do, the comfort stops too. Overeating is a habit seemingly beyond control.

The good news is that you are innocent of causing this habit. Your eating-for-comfort habit became established through no fault of your own: You were trained or programmed from birth to eat that way by well-meaning parents – especially mother. And it wasn't your mother's fault either. She acquired it from her mother who acquired it from hers, etc. So any guilt you may be harboring can now be let go; can now be thrown out the window of your mind. But regardless of your innocense, it does remain your responsibility to correct this erroneous program. Let's look at how this "conditioning" started and of what it consists.

The Primal Need for Security

Our feeling safe, secure and comfortable is the foundation and primary factor motivating most all of our actions, behaviors and general pursuit of happiness. It's what drives us. We need a minimum level of security and comfort in all areas of life. We want to feel secure physically, mentally, emotionally, financially, and in our relationships with others. If we don't have this minimum level of security, we feel the negative emotions of stress, fear, depression, sadness, doubt, anxiety, worry, discontent, resentment, lack of confidence, self-esteem, etc.

Now, when you were in your mother's spa-like womb, you were as secure as one could imagine – all of your wants and needs fully and effortlessly provided for. But when you passed through the birth canal into the alien outside world, things abruptly and dramatically changed. You became the most *in*secure imaginable – from the bright lights, loud noises and cold temperature of the operating-room, from being grossly severed from mother's body, held upside down by a masked stranger and spanked till you turned purple.

There was nothing you could do but cry your heart and lungs out. You were soon returned to mother who snugly held you, gently rocked you, and then, to comfort you, she placed a warm breast or bottle into your mouth. Having something in your mouth did prevent you from crying, but it contained food! And food was the last thing you wanted at the time. All you wanted was to be held and rocked – because that was the closest experience of being back in the comfort and security of your mother's womb.

This scenario of being fed whenever you cried was repeated hundreds of times after birth. Whenever you cried, your mother assumed you were either uncomfortable or hungry. So she'd first check your diaper. If clean, she placed a breast or bottle into your mouth to feed and pacify you, and when something is put into your mouth, the instinctive reaction is to chew. But you weren't hungry all those times. Again, you just wanted to be held and rocked. The result: *You became conditioned to equate food with comfort and security!* You were innocently and inadvertently trained to eat for emotional comfort instead of for physical nourishment.

Now this wasn't much of an issue in early childhood. You were quite comfortable in your warm, cozy home with your loving parents, caring siblings and fluffy dog. But then you had to leave that comfort zone. You had to leave another secure womb. This time to attend school and relate with unfamiliar boys, girls and teachers, study difficult material, pass grueling tests and compete in rigorous sports activities. All very stressful stuff. So you reacted in the way you were trained to react in uncomfortable situations – you headed to the refrigerator for some relief.

The subtle deception about this condition is that food really *does* comfort you, but it's a falsely-based, temporary and symptomatic comfort that stops the moment you stop eating – so, you don't want to stop eating. This is not the *real* you, not the *original,* healthy, self-controlled you. You were not born to overeat, not born to eat for stress relief, not born to be controlled by your appetite.

Overeating is not a genetically-transmitted disease. Food, in and of itself, is not an addictive substance. This overeating complex is something you acquired, and regardless of how acquired, it can be dropped starting the moment you realize, with the help of your mirror, your bathroom scale, and your cholesterol and blood pressure levels, that it's no longer serving you, that there's something wrong with this picture, something you now want to correct.

That your program is *subconscious* explains why it's so difficult to stop overeating, why you feel virtually powerless over food, why you cannot reason yourself thinner no matter how intelligent you are, no matter how much you try. Your appeals go in one ear and out the other. The subconscious mind is below the level of normal awareness, out of reach of conscious, reasoned control. This program continues to feel, remember, and believe that food relieves your stress, so, any attempt by your logical *conscious* mind to change things is going to be stubbornly hindered or blocked.

Think of this block as a security guard complex whose job is to "protect" you by *keeping* you eating for the wrong reason, *keeping* you eating in the erroneous way it was trained. The question becomes, how do you correct this erroneous program? How do you unblock, unbrainwash this part of you? How do you reverse or neutralize this emotional attachment, this illicit love affair with food?

Neutralizing Your Eating-for-Comfort Habit (ECH)

Now you didn't overeat in a vacuum. You didn't overeat with your mouth alone. Your thoughts, feelings and consciousness (or lack thereof) were involved as well. Effective and lasting recovery is an integrated, holistic package. To control one part of you, you have to control all parts of you. Otherwise you'd be treating the symptom, not the cause, and never reach your goal. Again, if attachment to your ECH has caused you to gain weight, then detaching from it will cause you to lose that weight. The way you reverse or neutralize the attachment is by cultivating the discipline of thinking all your thoughts, feeling all your feelings, and eating all your food, from a *conscious and respectable distance.* You think, feel and eat, not personally, but as if you were an impartial spectator, witness or outside observer.

This "distance" or space *is* the reality-based, appetite-controlling factor. It *is* the program-nullifying and neutralizing factor. You can't read a newspaper if held directly against your eyes; you have to "back off" a bit in order get the clarity and power to read. You have to get as if one step removed from it.

Detachment gives you the clarity to know when your body is

satisfied along with the power to stop right then and there. You then eat only for physical nourishment and no longer for emotional nourishment. You stop eating when the body is satisfied not when the emotions are satisfied, so it becomes virtually impossible to overeat. You want to cultivate a strictly "platonic" relationship with food; that is, you want your relationship with food to be physical and sensual – *not* emotional.

Respect the Integrity of the Relationship

The word "respectable" in this formula and context, means respecting the integrity of the relationship, respecting that it *is* a relationship – of two separate and distinct entities – your *awareness*, plus the food of which your awareness is aware. Awareness is not to be contaminated or diminished by the food the eyes are seeing, the food the nose is smelling, or the food the mouth is tasting.

Just as the ears can hear from some distance, the eyes can see from some distance, the nose can smell from some distance – *so can the mouth feel and taste from some a distance!* The ears actually are *apart* from the sounds they hear; the eyes actually are *apart* from the food it sees; the nose is actually *apart* from the aromas it smells – so is the mouth actually *separate* from the food it feels and tastes! All you have to do is to *consciously* keep them that way. Keep them separate – in their correct and "lawful" relationship. That's what detachment is and that's the primary discipline for you to cultivate.

Let's look at how your mind/body/spirit faculties are related to each other and to appetite control: You have seven lower faculties and one higher faculty. The seven lower, consist of your thoughts, feelings and five-senses. The higher "spiritual" faculty is non-other than your everyday, waking "consciousness," the part that's *aware* of the lower faculties thinking, feeling and eating. And it is by virtue of its transcendent, "above" position, that it controls your thinking, feeling and eating. You are conscious of your thoughts when you think them; therefore, your consciousness is in control of your thoughts. It's the same with your physical movements, emotional feelings, and sensual eating. Your consciousness is above them, therefore in control of them. It's your sixth sense or master sense. It's like the father/mother controlling their seven children.

Here is the problem restated: When you're eating from your "program" you're not eating from full consciousness – so there's little or no control. It's like the parent is absent and the children run wild, or like your seven pets have become unleashed. When eating from your program, you're eating only physically, mentally, emotionally and sensually. Your higher consciousness, your very source of clarity and power, is virtually absent from the equation, absent from the experience. You overeat because there's insufficient awareness to inform you of satiety and insufficient power to stop you.

A poem by Louisa May Alcott states the matter more succinctly:

> *"A little kingdom I possess*
> *Where thoughts and feelings dwell,*
> *And very hard the task I find,*
> *Of governing it well."*

Detachment brings your higher consciousness, your higher power, back into the picture, back into its correct and rightful position of supremacy over the lower faculties, back into "mind over matter." Detachment is a backward movement – away from the impotent lower, and toward the powerful higher. You become a centered personality, a centered eater.

The Three Levels of Eating

Now there are three levels of awareness while eating. The lowest level is virtually unconscious eating. That's when you eat, for example, while watching TV, reading, working, driving, etc. You're eating with so little awareness that you don't know you've had enough until it's too late, until you've overeaten by hundreds, even thousands of calories. And the worst part is, you're still hungry! It's like a big dog that swallows the whole can of food in one quick gulp, then quizzically looks up as if to say, "Is that it? Where's my meal? You call that dinner?" He's never satisfied because he never really tastes his food nor is aware whether he's full. And without awareness of satiety there's also no power to stop. Knowledge is power – stopping power.

The second level of eating is *emotional* eating. Again, you eat because it makes you *feel* better. You eat to relax tension or stress. You use food as a palliative to relieve some negative emotion such as boredom, resentment, doubt, fear, uncertainty, etc. And when anything makes you feel good, you want to continue it. Not only do you not want to stop, you become hardly able to stop. You become virtually powerless over food. With unconscious eating you don't know when you've had enough; with emotional eating, you not only don't know you've had enough, you don't care either; and even when you do care, you still can't stop.

Here again the higher consciousness is virtually absent from the eating equation, leaving you without clarity and power as well. You're disconnected from it. Devoid of it. You're like a kitchen toaster that's not plugged into its source or power, so can't achieve its intended purpose, can't fulfill its toast-making potential. The mental faculty is *only* for thinking. The emotional faculty is *only* for feeling. The sensual faculties are *only* for sensing. None of these lower faculties have intelligence or knowledge of their own. They all need higher consciousness in order to know and control what they're thinking, feeling and eating.

Consciousness is *above* thinking, feeling and eating, so your whole purpose here is to reach that state of "aboveness" and stay there. Detachment is how you get above and beyond them, how you get conscious, how you get control, how you get real, how you get healthier, happier and slimmer. The third and highest level of eating is the opposite of the lowest level. It's eating with full consciousness.

Now you may "think" you eat consciously, but consciousness comes in many degrees. If you're overweight, that's clear and incontrovertible evidence that your awareness level is low. And the way to raise awareness, again, is to get some distance from the senses sensing the food you're eating. Separate yourself from it. You can't read a newspaper held directly against your eyes, can you? You have to back off a little. You have to make a *space.* This space is necessary to see, to enlightenment, to clarity. The same with conscious eating, you have to get some distance from the food in order to get first-hand knowledge of satiety and its consequent stopping power. Detachment and consciousness are directly reciprocal: You can't be one without the other. You can't be more aware unless more detached, and vice versa.

The Law of Detachment Method (LDM) of Appetite-Control

The method of controlled eating consists of three overlapping phases: The first phase is to *eat slowly and from a conscious and respectable distance.* It's treating food more as a material object than as something personal. In a healthy relationship you wouldn't treat a person as an object – that would be demeaning. But conversely, you *do* want to treat food as an object. Food is not personal; people are. Treating food personally – meaning emotionally, is demeaning yourself. You're lowering yourself by elevating food. Food is just food. It doesn't have feelings and shouldn't affect feelings. Its purpose is physical and sensual satiety, not emotional satiety.

The second phase, *while* eating, is to remain acutely aware, like a Samurai warrior, of the very first sense that the hunger you began eating with has subsided. Notice that you're *not* eating until full or till you feel better – by then it's too late. That's the incorrect, programmed way you ate in the past. You're *eating only until the hunger has abated.* This happens when you've eaten about one-third to one-half your former meal size. Sometimes the hunger abates after just a few forkfuls of food – proving your body wasn't as hungry as you "thought." Eating is not a time for thinking; it's a time for *knowing,* a time for objective awareness.

Phase three is then to put that fork down and immediately *stop eating!* Reducing the method to twelve words, it's – *eat with slow detachment, watch for the hunger to subside, then stop!* That's it. Deceptively simple. Immensely powerful – especially when practiced in conjunction with Portion Control, which we'll discuss in the next chapter.

You eat when hungry then stop when the body is no longer

hungry, but the body will stop being hungry on a small fraction of your usual meal size. Pounds drop in due course without stress, willpower or undue feelings of deprivation. Food is no longer an issue in your life. The fact is this: *It's virtually impossible to overeat when you eat with a detachment.* You know clearly when the body is sated, and you powerfully stop right then. Clarity and appetite-control power go hand in hand. You are now in control of your mind and body, savoring every meal objectively, dispassionately, impersonally. You now eat like a gourmet, not like a glutton. Eating is now a meaningful, intimate experience – again, physically and sensually intimate, not emotionally intimate. You eat with reverence now. You eat with appreciation and gratitude now. You are not just feeding your face; you are deliciously nourishing your sacred, slimmer, healthier body. You now treat eating as meditation. In fact, you make it meditation – like the Japanese Tea Ceremony, for example.

Practicing LDM at a Restaurant

If you can eat detachedly at a restaurant with its myriad distractions, you'll easily be able to eat detachedly at home. Imagine that you and two friends are entering a restaurant, perhaps one of your favorite Italian restaurants, for a nice leisurely dinner – you, of course, now try to eat *all* your meals in a leisurely rather than rushed manner regardless of whether home alone or out with others.

You use the entrance to the restaurant as a device for entering detachment mode. Your stepping over the threshold triggers it. The smiling hostess seats you at a corner booth and hands you the parchment-paper menu. You detachedly notice how elegant the crispy paper feels in your hands.

You witness the olfactory sense begin to awaken as the distinctive and attractive smell of pungent garlic permeates the room. You open the starched, white cotton napkin and place it on your lap. The impatient new waiter arrives for your order before you've even opened the menu, but it doesn't disturb you as it would have in the past. In the past you'd have become upset and resentful over it. You'd have carried on a diatribe in your mind about what an incompetent oaf is this waiter – then you'd proceed to eat twice as much food as planned. You quickly recover yourself because you left home *anticipating* such glitches would occur.

You order the *Eggplant Parmigiana*. The group agrees on a bottle of Sangiovese wine. The eyes see a rosy pink carnation at the center of the round table and the nose smells its sweet perfume. The ears hear opera singing in the background. Sounds like Pavarotti or Boccelli. The volume is a bit too loud, though. A little disconcerting – proving you let yourself get caught up in the sound rather than remain above it. The volume should be so set that diners can tune it in or out at will. Normally you'd complain to management, but you're a different person now. You understand that resentment and judgment – all negative emotions, are fattening; all will trigger your ECH. You accept life – and restaurants, on their terms. You let things pass now. Maintain your poise. Practice a little tongue control. Don't think anything more of it. Becoming more confident and proud of yourself now.

The ears detachedly hear the busy, quiet din of about forty other diners in the room. The ambience is relaxed and pleasant – just like you always are now – well, almost always. Progress not perfection is your watchword. The initial sounds and smells serve both as sensual appetizers and as a reminder to not allow anything to distract you from your super-conscious eating agenda.

Soon the waiter places the plate in front of you – from the wrong side of course. You pause and take a deep breath. Then the eyes witness the entree you've chosen. You've ordered this dish many times, but now it's as if seeing it for the very first time. How visually appealing its appearance and presentation. The eyes witness the shapes and sizes of all the items – placed in so balanced and symmetrical a pattern. The eyes relish how vivid and varied the colors. It's a work of art. Just the sight of it causes salivation to begin. And you remember that it's not "you" seeing the food; it's the *eyes* seeing the food. The "you" remains above and distinct from the eyes seeing the food. And that's exactly the separation that gives you your increased clarity, power and slimmer body.

You then briefly close those delighted eyes and say silently but firmly to yourself the words, *slow and detached*. You open your eyes, mentally prepared to eat slowly and from a conscious *distance*. Slowly and from a *respectable* distance. You are respecting both the food and your sacred body. Everything's as if in silent, slow motion now. You're caught up as if in a reverie of present-moment super-consciousness. The hands pick up the knife and fork noticing how heavy and nicely engraved they are. You watch the hands cut a small morsel of the steaming, mozzarella-covered eggplant. You're sure it'd be all right, etiquette-wise, to cut two pieces at a time – but that'd be contrary to your slow-eating strategy. You return the knife to the plate and transfer the fork to your right hand – purposely using the American zigzag method rather than the Continental . Though less efficient, it's more conducive to controlled, deliberate eating. You slowly lift the eggplant straight up, then into the mouth. Then you return the fork to the plate and return your hand to your knee. The hand does not put more food into the mouth until the previous portion has been completely chewed and swallowed. You eat this mindfully even when alone – especially when alone.

The mouth chews very, very slowly, twenty, thirty, or forty times, depending on the density of the food, because you know it takes *time* for the stomach to inform the brain that it's had enough. There's no need to rush. The restaurant won't close for hours. You take twice as long to eat half as much. Your digestive system thanks you as it can now process the food easier and more efficiently. Even the lungs breathe easier. You're eating at just the right pace, at just the right rate.

The waiter comes over to refill the water glasses. He picks up the glasses with his fingers around the rim – where you put your mouth. What a dork! You start chewing like mad – because now you're angry. You stuff a huge forkful of linguine into your mouth, then another, then another. Your cheeks blow up like a squirrel. You soon catch yourself. You stop, take a deep breath, calm down. The old you would have carried the resentment all evening – and overeaten by a few thousand calories – not that you count calories. You don't ever have to do that again. For the rest of the meal, you drink your water with a straw. It's settled. You're never too old to grow up.

You maintain detached attention to eating while you're talking. Martha asks if you've become vegetarian because of your eggplant choice. You say you've been thinking about it. Jackie says her definition of a vegetarian is someone who doesn't eat meat unless someone else is paying for it. Everyone laughed – but you couldn't help wondering if she was referring to you, as you're sometimes accused of being frugal to a fault.

Martha says, "I'm on a seafood diet – I see food and I eat it." The laughter continues as the waiter empties the wine bottle into their glasses.

Then Jackie says, "You know, the trouble with eating Italian food is that five or six days later you're hungry again."

You maintain eating awareness through the laughter. The mouth gently caresses the food. The tongue moves the food from side to side and back and forth, and round and round on the tongue, cheeks, palate, lips and teeth. The sharp, front incisors bite into the food, then the cuspids chew it into small pieces. The bicuspids break up and crush the course food while the multi-surfaced molars in back do most of the chewing. You want to get the very most benefit from every single morsel, to not miss the tiniest iota of delicious flavor.

The mouth is eating less but enjoying it so much more. The mouth detachedly *feels* the hot or cold temperature and the smooth and crunchy textures of the food, as thousands of happy little taste buds now burst open to begin savoring a circus of delightful flavors and aromas. You watch the mouth taste how sweet or sour, how salty or bitter, how spicy or bland, how sharp or mild, how pungent or delicate, how juicy and succulent. You *witness* the salivation and gentle swallowing as the solids become almost liquid. Mahatma Ghandi said, "You should drink your food and eat your water."

Pausing between bites to discern whether or not the body is sated, you slowly reach over and grasp the bowl of your wine glass and lift it to the mouth. Stopping to sip the wine or water gives you a perfect opportunity to feel whether the body is yet sated. You *honestly* decide it isn't. You lift the glass to eye level and swirl it around a bit. The eyes see its brownish, mahogany color, and how fast the legs streak down the glass. You notice how the bouquet reaches the nose before the glass touches the lips. The nose sniffs the wine – first from a little distance, then you put the nose deep into the glass to notice an earthy, herbal aroma – perhaps black cherry. You heard that taste is eighty-percent smell. The lips pucker up, take a sip, and swirl it around in the mouth to expose it to all the taste buds. The full body, smoothness and dryness are the first impressions on the palate. The throat swallows now and you detachedly notice the remnants of the aftertaste on the back of the throat. The taste lingers to embellish the next bite of food.

While you're eating, awareness remains *undistractedly* rooted in the present moment, immediately noticing when that awareness wanders or the conversation distracts you, then you return intimate, dispassionate, platonic attention to the delicious, nourishing food.

You find that you can converse and eat detachedly at the same time. You can do two things at the same time. And you remember that it's not "you" tasting the food; it's the *taste buds* that taste the food, while it's the higher you, the conscious you, the powerful you, the slimmer you – that *witnesses* the taste buds tasting the food. Thus the "you" remains above and distinct from the food. The "you" remains aloof from the food. The "you" remains above it all. Separate from the food. The "you" are one step removed from the food. The "you" are no longer caught up in food, no longer engrossed in food. The "you" no longer eats emotionally. The "you" now eats mindfully, impersonally – from reality, clarity, power, healthfulness and slimness. You are not just eating; you are intensely *aware* that you're eating. You know that you know you're eating.

And all while, that "witness" of yours, that sixth sense, that all-controlling master sense remains acutely aware, like a cat at a mouse-hole, for the very first inkling that the hunger has subsided – then you *stop eating immediately!* The body is finished eating. The hand returns the fork to the plate for the last time, and you're delighted to notice that the body is fully sated on a third of the food on that plate. How wonderful! The emotional attachment is broken. The mental obsession is lifted. The obstruction is removed. Deliverance has come.

Then you rest awhile in pleased satisfaction and gratitude – gratitude that you are now in control of food and that no longer does food control you. And with a big inner smile of pride and joy, you have the server those leftovers to enjoy later. How sweet it is to be finally free. You feel good about your life now, and the pounds drop as planned, never to return.

Words that rhyme are easier to remember, so the following poem should make it easier for you to memorize the *Law of Detachment Method:*

"I enjoy four portion-controlled meals per day,

Eating in a slow and detached way;

Watching for the hunger to subside,

Then stopping for that is my guide!"

Overcoming Anorexia and Bulimia

It's normal human nature to want to improve, fix or change something about your looks – like to become thinner. But when that common desire becomes an obsession that dominates your life, then you've crossed the line toward a serious physical, mental or emotional health problem.

So far, we've been discussing compulsive overeating in general. Let's turn now to the less common, but more unhealthy and dangerous eating disorders: *Anorexia and Bulimia.* What are they and how can they be effectively treated using the *Law of Detachment Method*?

Anorexia nervosa is a Greek term meaning "lack of appetite." It's defined as excessive weight loss by excessive fasting or deliberate self-starvation. The anorexic has an intense or morbid fear of getting fat even though she may be underweight. This is a self-developed *habit* and not a disease, per se, but it's as insidious as alcoholism in that it gradually and subtly progresses to debilitating levels.

Bulimia Nervosa, also from the Greek, means "Eating like an ox." It's characterized by repeated, secretive episodes of binge eating followed by purging – as a means of controlling weight. Purging is the evacuation of the bowels – getting rid of the food, usually by self-induced vomiting or diarrhea. Methods include abusing laxatives, diuretics, enemas, diet pills, over-exercising and fasting.

The approach to overcoming these disorders, or any variation of them, is two-fold – stopping the behavior, then staying stopped. First, you'll apply *The Law of Detachment Method* to the every nuance of the anorexic/bulimic episode – as described earlier for the compulsive overeater; then, the maintenance phase is to follow the methods of the *Appetite Control, Portion Control, and Stress Control* methods described in this and subsequent chapters. These methods work by replacing the unwanted habit/program with a healthy one.

The theory behind the power of the LDM, again, is that any unwanted behavior that's *consciously* experienced to the end, can and will be terminated at will. The premise is that during the bulimarexic experience you are in a virtual trance, and objective awareness is the means by which to break that trance. (See the fuller explanation in the *Introduction*.) The law can't fail; only the operator can fail through inexperience. So if it doesn't work the first or second time, keep practicing till it does. The two disorders sufficiently overlap in their symptoms so that we can treat them together using the commonly-used term, *bulimarexic*.

Applying the LDM to Bulimarexia

Here you'll apply the method in your imagination. In daily activity, you'll apply it to the actual bulimarexic experience or episode. You'll *observe* your thoughts, feelings and actions as you go about your day to the best of your ability Using your imagination will help you to practice the detached perspective. A good "distancing" technique is to imagine yourself sitting in front of a large movie screen *witnessing* yourself going through your day. The idea is to have, *as if*, an "out of body" experience of it, so that you can see what you're doing with such clarity that it will break your identity with it, break your attachment to it, break your love affair with it, break the vicious cycle of it. Not all aspects of the following guided example will apply to you, but you'll get the point and benefit just the same.

See yourself awaking in the morning. You look at yourself in the mirror. Notice what do you think and feel about how you look? You notice everything now, how often you look in the mirror and how often you weigh yourself and what you think of the readings. You notice at what point the thought of food or eating first enters your mind.

You're always on a strict diet – which, you now notice, usually triggers the binge/purge cycle. You didn't pre-plan breakfast. You see yourself look in the refrigerator and decide on one fried egg, one slice of dry whole wheat toast, a half-cup of non-fat cottage cheese and a black coffee. You count the calories, carbohydrates and fat. You sit at the table and watch yourself methodically cut your egg into eight small pieces. You also cut the toast into eight pieces.

You eat fast to get it over with. The egg tastes good and you think of spitting it out. You got the taste, so what do you need the fat for? But you do swallow it, and with that first swallow, like the alcoholic's first drink, you just know that this isn't going to be enough. The cottage cheese tastes awful. You think of adding honey to it but immediately dismiss the idea.

Your husband leaves for work and asks if that's all you're going to eat. You know why he asked that question and know that he'll not be able to put up with this behavior for much longer. You tell him you're going to have some pancakes too, but don't have them. After he leaves, you open the pancake box and dump a cup of mix down the drain. You continue eating mindlessly till about half-way through the meal, then abruptly throw the rest into sink, and run the disposal for several minutes to get rid of the smell.

You think you've eaten too much and hurry to change into jogging gear. You jog three miles at a faster than usual speed. Your heart-rate monitor tells you to slow down, but that half egg and slice of toast had so much fat, you decide to run even longer and faster. You get home, do some strenuous weight-lifting and stretching exercises, then shower and weigh yourself again.

You observe that the tension and craving for more food has already begun – the second phase of the vicious cycle after eating a severely limited meal. You repeat this routine with lunch – though you think you should have skipped lunch after eating so much at breakfast.

You notice the stress and craving continuing through the afternoon. You know your husband won't be home for dinner, so you begin thinking about what you'll eat. It'll be more than you had for breakfast or lunch – that's for sure.

You've been feeling a little sad and lethargic lately. You're home alone and bored. You're getting a little sick and tired of this battle, this constant struggle between binging and fasting. You really don't want to binge. You know you'll feel terrible afterwards, but you always do it anyway. You watch yourself put on some baggy clothes to cover what you think is an unattractive body, and drive to the supermarket. You didn't "plan" dinner, so you fill the cart with a variety of items so that your choices won't be limited come dinnertime. You hope no one you know sees all the food in your cart.

You watch yourself hurrying home and quickly putting away the food. You put the 18-ounce frozen lasagna in the microwave for ten-minutes. At about seven-minutes through, you'll add an extra layer of mozzarella cheese on top. You start frying the four Italian sausages in garlic and olive oil, and heat up three French rolls.

You place the completed meal in front of you and light a candle –

add some dignity to your pig out. At this point, you notice yourself going into a kind of trance mode. Time seems to stand still. Your mind closes. Nothing exists now but the food. You start eating, slowly at first, then a little faster. You witness yourself keep eating, and eating and eating. You don't chew the food very well as you want to slow the digestion process. You soon feel your stomach is filled to capacity but you ignore it and keep eating. You didn't leave room for dessert, but you'll have some anyway. While stilling chewing the sausage, you warm up a quarter of apple-cinnamon pie and add two scoops of French vanilla ice cream. You finish it before the ice cream melts too much.

The binge is over. Now the panic sets in. You have to undo this 4,000-calorie binge. Now comes the purging, the forth phase of the cycle: You see yourself hurry to the toilet, take a triple dose of laxatives, and fall to your knees with your head inside the bowl. You force two fingers deep into your throat and start throwing up. You keep vomiting until no more will come out. You sit on the bowl until the diarrhea has finished flowing. You flush the toilet several times, then brush it with bleach. You spray the toilet with deodorant to hide the awful smell of vomit before your husband comes home. You gargle some mouthwash and chew some breath mints.

You come out of the trance now – with the usual feelings of disgust, shame and guilt – the fifth and last phase of the cycle. You think of the lost time, energy and health, the self-loathing, the stolen dignity and self-respect.

There's a few moments of silence, then a realization comes to you, a wonderfully simple idea that never occurred to you before – that you don't ever have to do this again, that it's over, that it's okay to not do this again. You know now that you have the power to stop doing it and that you've always had the power. You just didn't know it before; now you do. You've broken the vicious cycle. The obsession has been removed. It's perfectly clear now that you *can* eat in a normal, natural, self-controlled way.

You smile with gratitude as the self-hate turns to self-love and self-respect. The shame and guilt are replaced by innocence; the sadness by joy; the anxiety by peace of mind; the bondage by freedom; the fear by supreme confidence.

Key Points and Principles to Remember from Chapter 2:

1. That being overweight is a condition in which the appetite controls you instead of you controlling the appetite;

2. That you were habituated during infancy to eat for emotional comfort and security;

3. That this wrong purpose and relationship with food leads to eating disorders such as binge or compulsive overeating, anorexia and bulimia;

4. That this habit/behavior is rooted in the subconscious mind and can't be controlled until it's made *conscious*;

5. That this habit is made conscious by witnessing every aspect of the eating experience/behavior from a *conscious distance,* and noting the exact moment the hunger has subsided (The Law of Detachment Method);

6. That all thoughts and feelings are also controlled by keeping a *conscious distance* from them.

CHAPTER 3

HOW TO CONTROL YOUR PORTIONS

"You don't have to have a brain; you just have to know the road." – Scarecrow, *The Wizard of Oz*

The Plan is The Thing

The last chapter spoke of *how* to eat; this chapter deals with the nuts and bolts of what, why, when and how much to eat. Regulating food portions is the third of the five steps toward nullifying your eating-for-comfort habit.

The first step – *Recreating your self-image*, gives your subconscious a model to copy or recreate; the second step – *appetite control via detachment*, causes hunger to be sated on smaller amounts of food, while *portion-control* helps prevent eating *beyond* that point. The idea is this: If there's no food left on your plate, you can't eat it.

You've noticed that "The spirit is willing but the flesh is weak." Portion control is the natural way to support the spirit and overcome the flesh. Just as you wouldn't take medications and dosages not prescribed by your doctor, so you wouldn't choose foods and portions sizes not prescribed by your plan. Your plan becomes the leader; your body, the follower. The plan, in and of itself, is virtually more important than its contents – for if you give method to your madness, it's no longer madness. The mental, physical and emotional become subservient to your plan. They are *already* subservient to a plan – but to a fattening or bulimarexic plan. So what you're doing here is simply replacing an unconscious, erroneous plan with a conscious, healthy one.

Most of your day is already conducted by plan: Rising at a certain time and way; getting the children off to school in a certain way; getting to work on time, by a certain route, then working all day according to a plan prescribed by the "job description," etc. Daily food planning should be no less a natural, integral, routine part of your day – at least equal in importance to all other activities in your day. And if you want to lose weight, then it should take an even higher priority than most other activities. So food planning isn't really a choice; it's mandatory – an integral part of the Law of Detachment's creative self-control process. Remember that "failing to plan is planning to fail." Get in the habit of doing everything "by the numbers" like the military does – which is the discipline that's key to their great power.

Weigh and Measure

Weighing and measuring food in advance prevents, first, the sensual *temptation* to continue eating – "I know I'm full but it's so tasty, I'll keep eating anyway!" And second, weighing and measuring prevents the build-up of *momentum* of the physical eating process – a mouth in motion tends to stay in motion.

The purpose of portion-control is to remove personal discretion from the decision-making process. Left to your own devices (your

ECH), you'll always prepare and eat larger portions than your body wants or needs. Remember that your appetite or behavior is driven by your subconscious program, not the logical, rational, intelligent part of your mind. So the amount of food you "think" you need will always be either excessive of deficient depending on your disorder. Your thoughts, feelings and eyes will always be bigger than your stomach; therefore, you can't trust those faculties in this matter. Your eating life, then, will need to be more specifically prescribed and organized than it is now.

Even though you're replacing a bad habit with a good one, it will still feel awkward in the beginning, as all new habits do. Be patient. It only takes about twenty-one to thirty days for a new habit to become assimilated. Once it has, you'll feel very proud of yourself for having acquired it, and gained power over your life.

The Freedom of Limitation

Portion-control won't be as burdensome or stifling as it may sound. In fact, it'll be quite the opposite. It will be more liberating because you won't have to think about food all the time. You won't need to obsess about it any longer. Your eating life will be settled in advance, so you can forget about it and go on with other areas of your life. This will free you up to get a life – a life beyond food. Portion control adds rhyme and reason to your eating. It frees you by limiting you.

Limitation doesn't mean the loss of spontaneity and creativity. On the contrary, it fosters and stimulates them. An artist works within the limitations of her medium or canvas. She chooses to work on a 16" by 20" canvas, for example. That size is her "limitation," but within it, her choice of subject and style is unlimited – or limited only by her imagination. The same with your food planning. You're limited to a certain number of balanced meals and certain amounts food, but within those strictures you can be as spontaneous and creative as you'd like.

Eat Four Times a Day

Your structured eating plan begins with enjoying four meals a day – breakfast, lunch, dinner, and a mini-meal. Eating four times a day means eating about every four hours. For example, at about 8:00, 12:00, 4:00, and 7:00 P.M. – modified, of course, to accommodate your individual work, social and sleep schedule. Setting your cell phone alarm to sound every four hours will further simplify the matter. Eating four times a day keeps the fat-burning metabolism running on high. Eating more frequent, smaller meals will also prevent you from feeling hungry throughout the day.

Do the same with water: drink a glass of pure, clear, uncolored water *every hour*. This will free your body from the need to retain fluids. It will wash away fatty toxins and cellulite. It will make you feel more refreshed and energized, and will diminish between-meal cravings. Many cravings for food are actually a thirst for water.

You should eat breakfast within one-hour of waking because your metabolism has slowed during the night, and breakfast will rev it up again. You should also have your mini-meal at least three-hours before bedtime so your food can fully digest before then. Going to sleep with a full stomach makes it easier for fat to establish a storage space – especially around the mid-section. Another caveat is that digestion uses lots of energy which may also interfere with the quality of your sleep. And a good night's sleep is integral to good health in general and waking refreshed and energized in particular.

And finally, you should eat *nothing* between meals – not even a celery stick! This is key to greatly diminishing between-meal cravings. Here's why: When you eat something, even something as innocent as a grape, for example, it signals the salivary glands, stomach and small intestine to start releasing about twenty-two digestive enzymes and acids to help with the digestion and absorption process. All systems are go, and they anticipate and *expect* more food to come down. No more food is coming but they wait and wait and wait; and this waiting is *felt* as a craving for food. But the body is not necessarily hungry! You simply tempted and excited the digestive system with that innocent grape!

Determine Correct Portion Size

The "correct" portion sizes for you will differ depending on whether you're in the temporary phase of losing weight, or in the lifelong phase of maintaining your goal weight. During the maintenance phase of eating, the particular amount of food that caused the hunger to subside will be the correct portion. For example, if you were eating a meal in the slow and detached way prescribed by the First Step, and noticed the hunger abated at about sixteen-ounces of a balanced meal, then, all other things being equal, sixteen-ounces would be the correct portion size for you. The idea is this: You want the plate to become empty at the same time the hunger subsides. Then you are simply eating when hungry and stopping when no longer hungry. You would naturally eat just enough to maintain your desired weight indefinitely. The same principle applied to your financial planning might be to die and run out of money at same time.

If you're still in the weight-*losing* phase, however, you'll have to eat less than the sixteen ounces. You'd have to eat only ten or twelve ounces in order to reduce your weight (or exercise more).

The following Weight-Reduction Plan should help take the guesswork out of it for you. As one size doesn't fit all, this is just a general guideline. Again, following a portion-control plan is more important than what the portion amounts are. The portions/serving sizes given here are for women. Men may add one or two ounces of protein and starch per meal.

It will be useful to remember that your stomach is about the size of a closed fist, and many portions sizes are about the size of the palm of your hand. Weighing and measuring everything will soon become an enjoyable, effective habit. It will give you a warm feeling of pride that comes with being more in control of your life.

Sample Weight Reduction Plan

BREAKFAST: 3 oz. protein (3 servings), 4 oz. starch/grain (1 serving), 6 oz/1 cup fruit serving (1 serving), 1 cup dairy or substitute (1 serving).

LUNCH: 3 oz. protein (3 servings), 4 oz. starch/grain (1 serving), 6 oz./1cup fruit serving

(1 serving), 9 oz. vegetable (3 servings), 1 tbs. fat (2 servings).

DINNER: 4 oz. protein (4 servings), 4 oz. starch/grain (1 serving), 6 oz./1cup fruit serving (1 serving), 9 oz. vegetable (3 servings), 1 tbs. fat (2 servings).

MINI-MEAL: 4 oz. starch/grain (1 serving), 6 oz/1cup fruit serving (1 serving), 1 cup dairy or substitute (1 serving).

It should be pointed out here that satiety supersedes any food plan: If while eating according to the method the hunger subsides before the plate is empty, then you'd stop eating immediately, even though the "plan" says you're "allowed" more. The intuitive wisdom of your mind/body is always superior to external instructions. You just have to pay closer attention. Use leftovers as part of a subsequent meal, or give it to Fido, or throw it away. It's better to waste food than "waist" your body. This is good "waist" management. You're eating for health, happiness and freedom – not to save money. It's better to be a fat-pincher than a penny-pincher.

Portion and Serving Size

What's the difference between a portion size and a serving size? A serving size is a standard measurement of food – usually one that's recommended by the U.S. Food and Drug Administration (FDA). Serving size varies according to the food group. A portion is the *amount* of food you eat, which could consist of multiple servings.

Protein Group: 1 oz. = 1 serving (Lean meat, poultry, fish, cottage or ricotta cheese, eggs or egg substitute, beans, tofu, low fat hard cheese, soy burgers, milk, yogurt.)

Grains and Starchy Vegetables: 1 oz. = 1 serving (Bread, rice cake, potato, brown rice, oatmeal, non-sugared cereal, cream of wheat, corn, peas, winter squash, carrots, beets.)

Non-Starchy Vegetable Group: 1 cup = 2 servings (Asparagus, broccoli, celery, eggplant, greens, mushrooms, peppers, tomatoes, turnip, zucchini, string beans, cucumber, etc.)

Fruit Group: 1 cup = 2 servings (Apple, orange, peach, plum, kiwi, banana, strawberry, cherries, watermelon, cantaloupe, prune, apricot.)

Dairy Group: 1 cup = 1 serving (Low- or non-fat milk, soy milk, yogurt, cheese.)

Fats & Oils: 1 teaspoon = 4 grams (Low fat margarine, butter, mayonnaise, salad dressing.)

1 tablespoon = 3 teaspoons = 15 ml.

1 cup = 16 tablespoons = 240 ml.

1 ounce = 28.35 grams

Weight Maintenance Plan

Once you've reached your desired weight, you may change to a balanced maintenance plan such as the one suggested below. Here are some general guidelines for the number of daily servings suggested from each food group.

Grains and Starchy Vegetables Group: 6-11 servings a day/1 oz. = 1 serving

Non-Starchy Vegetable Group: 3-5 servings a day/1 cup = 2 servings

Dairy Group: 2-4 servings a day/1 cup = 1 serving

Meat and Beans Group: 4-6 servings a day/1 oz. = 1 serving

Fruit Group: 2-3 servings a day/1 cup = 2 servings

Fats & Oils: 24g or 6 teaspoons/1 teaspoon = 4 grams.

BREAKFAST: 4 oz. protein (4 servings), 6 oz/1 cup fruit serving (2 servings).

LUNCH: 4 oz. protein (4 servings), 1 cup cooked vegetable (1 serving), 1 cup raw vegetables or salad (1 serving), 2 tbs dressing.

DINNER: 4 oz. protein (4 servings), 1 cup cooked vegetable (1 serving), 2 cups raw vegetable (2 servings), 1 tbs. fat (2 servings).

MINI-MEAL: 2 oz. protein (2 servings), 6 oz/1cup fruit serving (2 servings), 1 cup dairy or substitute (1 serving).

The same caveat that applies to the Weight Reduction Plan applies to the Weight Maintenance Plan: Eat slowly and detachedly, while watching attentively for the hunger to subside, then stop – regardless of what the plan suggests or the amount of leftovers. Remember that it's always that last, illicit, impulsively eaten, seemingly innocent morsel of food that will foil your best-laid plans every time. So that's the one to watch out for.

Advance Meal Planning

A plan is a series of steps, thought out in *advance* of execution, to facilitate and ensure that the execution will be successful. If the plan works on paper, it is most likely to work in practice. If there's no plan, or the plan isn't followed, then your weight loss goal is unlikely to be achieved.

Step Three consists of three phases: *Weighing/Measuring, Advance Meal Planning, and Keeping a Journal*. This is a very powerful weight-management team, a reality-based, detachment-based team. There are three possible planning methods: You could plan meals for the entire week (28 meals) in advance; you could plan for the whole day (four meals) in advance; or plan each individual meal in advance. Research indicates the "one day at a time" approach is the most simple and effective because it aligns with the body's natural biorhythm, and because life does happen one day at a time. Build a wall around your day and eat and live within it. It makes shopping easier, too. It eliminates the disorder and risk of having to make choices on whim or while hungry. You could plan the night before or first thing in the morning, perhaps after you exercise, meditate and shower.

The efficacy of Advance Meal Planning is the same as for portion control. It removes mental and emotional considerations (your ECH) from the food-choosing and eating process. You eat according to nutritional needs rather than mood or caprice. There's nothing to think about; you just have to follow the instructions. Fat dissolves by itself. So remember the five P's: "Prior Planning Prevents Poor Performance."

Make a Hit List

It's also helpful to make a list of those foods that you know are not healthy and avoid them, especially those foods and ingredients that you know are your "trigger" or "binge" foods – those foods that you eat in large quantities or to the exclusion of other foods; foods that you turn to in times of celebration, sadness, stress or boredom; or foods that are high in calories and low in nutritional value. In addition, look to see whether there are any common ingredients among those foods – like refined sugar or fat that might exist in foods you haven't listed.

Below are examples of foods and eating behaviors that have been known to cause excessive cravings. Each of us may have problems with different foods or ingredients. If a food has been a binge food in the past, or if it contains ingredients that have been binge foods for you, remove it from your plan. For example, if pasta is a trigger food, then other foods made with flour (breads, muffins, crackers) could cause problems. Extra servings of a non-trigger food might create cravings. If you are unsure whether a food causes problems for you, leave it out at first.

Here are some examples: "Comfort" foods or junk foods such as chocolate, name-brand fast foods, cookies, potato chips. Foods containing refined sugar such as desserts, sweetened drink products and cereals, many processed meats, many condiments. Foods containing fats such as butter, cheese and other high-fat dairy or non-dairy foods, deep-fried foods and snacks, and many desserts. Foods containing wheat or flour or refined carbohydrates in general such as pastries, certain pastas and breads. Foods containing mixtures of sugar and fat, or sugar, flour and fat such as ice cream, doughnuts, cakes and pies. Foods you eat in large quantities even though they aren't your trigger foods.

When you identify the foods and ingredients that cause you cravings, you simply stop eating them. Remember that you are the boss of your body. As you practice patience, perseverance – and detached awareness, your interest in wrong foods and behaviors will leave you without effort or willpower. Remember that nothing tastes as good as being thinner feels.

Keeping a Journal

Keeping a record of what you eat and drink gives you perspective and objectivity. It helps you take a clear and critical look at your food habits when the concentrated action of eating is over. Writing down what you just ate allows you to deal with food in a relaxed, organized way. Your journal will help you to recognize why and when you eat the foods you do. And it will provide the means to discern the nutrient content and balance of your food.

Each day, note down *everything* that goes into your mouth – right after you eat it. You don't want to rely on memory because it's too convenient to "forget" eating the wrong food or amount at the wrong time. Be specific. And most important – be honest! Nothing is more slimming than honesty and integrity. It is the spiritual flavor that makes everything fall into place for you.

Slips will happen. When they do, simply note them down and think nothing of it. Never berate yourself. Remember that subconsciously you're *already* there. Slips will occur less and less frequently. Notice how time, place, situation and certain people you're with affect what and how much you ate. For instance, were you driving, watching TV, at work, at a restaurant, on a cruise, alone or with others. Notice your mood – angry, bored, tired, lonely, stressed, rushed, excited, etc. Notice, especially, that you tend to eat less and better food simply by virtue of recording it. Your journal becomes an angelic friend – warding off temptation and gently nudging you on the straight and narrow path toward your goal of health, beauty and freedom.

Rewarding Yourself

Your mind/body transformation will be its own reward, but till you get there, rewarding yourself along the way with a little pat on the back is highly motivating. Mary Kay Ash said, "There are 2 things people want more than sex or money – recognition and praise!" And recognition begins at home, so for each increment or short-term goal that is achieved, have a planned reward set up in advance. Here a some suggestions: Enjoy a day at the spa with a hot-rock massage and sauna; enjoy dinner at a fine French restaurant; buy a new (smaller) dress or exercise outfit; treat yourself to a night on the town; get a pedicure; go to a play or concert; buy a smoothie machine or a new cookbook; relax and enjoy a candle lit bubble bath with a bottle of Champagne, etc.

Key Points and Principles to Remember from Chapter 3:

1. The purpose of Portion Control is to remove (detach) all personal discretion from the decision-making process;

2. Pre-plan all meals, daily or weekly;

3. Weigh/measure all meals to prevent temptation and momentum;

4. Eat (with slow detachment) 4 times a day with nothing in between;

5. Drink a glass of water every hour;

6. List and avoid known binge or trigger foods;

7. Record/journal all meals to maintain awareness and objectivity;

8. Weigh yourself daily during the weight-loss phase, then weekly thereafter;

9. Reward your patient progress regularly.

CHAPTER 4

HOW TO EXERCISE YOUR BODY

"If you don't take care of your body, where will you live?"

Make a Commitment

Your subconscious now has a clear image of the body it is to create. That's the first step – the *creative* step; then you learned the two *eating* steps – controlling your appetite and controlling your portions. Physical exercise is the fourth interrelated step. These four, along with the Stress-Control comprise a total mind/body/spirit plan that is virtually infallible – but you have to do it. This is not a pill, a stomach-stapling, or any quick fix fantasy; it's a reality-based plan of disciplined *action* – which is the only thing that works long term. All you have to do is make it a habit – which psychologists say takes only about twenty-one to thirty days. Remember that good habits are just as addictive as bad habits.

The detachment-related elements of this method are ones you can easily practice for life. Now the idea of doing something for life may sound a little daunting – especially if you haven't yet habituated yourself to exercise and experienced the joy and power of it. To this end, it will be very helpful to not think in terms of a lifetime commitment, but to a *daily* commitment; a "one day at a time" attitude that we discussed earlier. You can practice all the steps in this method just one day at a time. You can do anything for just one day. You can stand on your head for just one day. So, again, build an imaginary wall around your day and live your whole healthier, happier, thinner life within it.

Commitment to regular physical activity is more important than the intensity of the workouts. Choose exercises you're likely to enjoy – ideally ones that are part of a sport or hobby like Tennis, Golf, Ballroom dance, etc. Progress slowly. Remember, it's not necessary to be exhausted to lose weight, and it's never too late to start exercising.

Making the decision to change your lifestyle, lose weight, and become healthier is a big step to take. It's helpful to put your commitment in writing – in the form of a contract with yourself. You've already "contracted" to lose a specific amount of weight by a specific date, in a specific way. Now you want to commit to a specific, well-thought-out exercise routine that works for you. It can be as simple or comprehensive as you'd like.

As the nature of the mind is to be still, the nature of the body is to move. The less the body moves the more muscles atrophy, lose tone and flexibility. Unexercised muscle groups attract fat like a magnet as metabolic rate slows and prevents the burning of that fat. Energy and vitality levels lower causing feelings of lethargy, lack of enthusiasm, apathy, mental and physical sluggishness, etc. One part of you drags down another part of you.

Physical activity works just the opposite – it improves the quality and character of every area of life. You think better, feel better, function better and look better. Scientifically established benefits include the following: Your heart, lungs and circulatory system become stronger. Blood pressure drops. Pulse rate slows down. Red blood cells increase. Energy increases. Digestion improves. Bowels function better. Appetite is brought into line with your body's needs. Weight loss is accelerated. Libido increases. Stress is reduced. Depression reverses. The level of high-density lipoproteins (HDL) increases – which help to keep fat from building up in the arteries.

The Physical-Activity Lifestyle

Now that you understand how important physical activity is to your health in general and weight loss in particular, the next step is incorporating it into your life. Do not feel overwhelmed by all this. It will be easier than you might think. In fact, you probably already are physically active and don't even know it. If you don't like to exercise right now, don't worry. Exercise is just one aspect of physical activity.

See if a friend would like to join you in your quest to lose weight and become more active. Things are a lot easier and more fun when a friend is involved too. Call your local Parks and Recreation Department, YMCA, or community organization to find out if they offer any programs or classes that may interest you. Many community centers and local colleges offer a variety of dance classes, exercise classes, yoga, aerobics, Tai Chi, cycling clubs, tennis lessons, swimming lessons, etc. Locate parks, and walking trails in your area. Local malls sometimes have walking clubs as well. It's a good place to go when the weather is bad.

Plan for the Week

Keep an activity journal. The journal can be separate from your eating journal or they can be combined. List all of the activities you have done or plan to do each day. A journal will help you track your progress and set goals. What has an exercise plan to do with detachment? Again, a plan removes personal discretion from the decision-making process. Use the Exercise Log in Appendix 5, or create your own. Track your exercise time and progress just as you record your meals. It helps you set your activity goals and stay on course. Before you know it, you'll be able to do at least 3 hours of moderate-level activities each week. Physical activity experts say that spreading aerobic activity out over at least three days a week is best. Also, do each activity for at least 20 minutes at a time. There are many ways to fit in 3 hours a week. For example, you can do 30 minutes of aerobic activity each day, for five days. On the other two days, do muscle-strengthening activities. Find what works for you. If you want to learn more about how to add physical activity to your life, join a fitness group. Talk to your health care provider about good activities to try, and search the Internet.

Reasons cited for not sticking to one's exercise program include lack of time, inconvenience, expense, physical discomfort, embarrassment, poor instruction, inadequate support, and loss of interest. These areas need to be addressed in order to maximize sticking to your plan. Time management is an important part of everyone's life and finding time to exercise is vital. According to the *American College of Sports Medicine* (ACSM) guidelines, workout time should be about 20 to 60 minutes, although this can be revised depending on whether an individual exercises more than 3-5 times a week or less than 3-5 times a week.

In scheduling your workout time it's important to allow time for travel, changing, showering, etc. If you're not relaxed or feel hurried when working out, you're less likely to enjoy your workout and so will be less likely to stick to your program.

 Be consistent in your program. Do it regularly every chosen day at the same time. This way you'll become psychologically and physiologically accustomed to the routine. Eventually your workout will become as habitual as showering. Don't skip more than one day. It's much too easy, particularly in the beginning, to go back to your old ways of sedentary, fat-storing, non-activity. Learn to love it and look forward to it every day with joyful anticipation. Hold the attitude that a day without exercise is like a day without sunshine.

Setting Realistic Goals

Set some short-term exercise goals and reward your efforts along the way. Focus on two or three goals at a time. Effective goals are specific, realistic, and forgiving. For example, "Exercise More"is not a specific goal. But if you say, "I will walk 30 minutes, Monday, Wednesday and Friday for the first week," you are setting a specific and realistic goal for the first week.

Small changes every day can lead to big results. Look for progress not perfection. Also remember that realistic goals are *achievable* goals. By achieving your short-term goals one day at a time, you'll feel good about your progress and be motivated to continue. Setting unrealistic goals will only leave you feeling defeated and frustrated.

Being realistic also means expecting occasional setbacks. Setbacks happen when you get away from your plan for whatever reason — maybe the holidays, longer work hours, or another life change. When setbacks happen, get back on track as quickly as possible. Also take some time to think about what you would do differently if a similar situation happens, to prevent setbacks. When you feel like giving up, remember why you held out so long in the first place.

Everyone is different – what works for someone else might not be right for you. Just because your neighbor lost weight by taking up running, doesn't mean running is the best option for you. Try a variety of activities – walking, swimming, tennis, or group exercise classes to see what you enjoy most and can fit into your life. These activities will be easier to stick with over the long term.

The Basic Physical Exercise Program

A well-rounded program of physical activity for weight loss will include *aerobic exercise, strength training exercise, and flexibility training*. These three types of exercise need not be done in the same session. Create a pattern or routine that you're comfortable with, that you'll stick to, and that fits into your schedule.

Aerobic Activity

Aerobic activity is anything that increases your breathing and heart rate. It involves continuous, rhythmic movement of large groups of muscles to strengthen your heart and lungs. In general, you should aim to do moderate-intensity activity for a minimum of 30 minutes, five days a week, or vigorous-intensity activity for 20 minutes, three days a week. You don't have to do the entire 20 or 30 minutes in one session to enjoy the benefits. For example, you can add up your activity by doing three sessions of 10 minutes or more.

It's better to exercise for a shorter period of time than not at all. Typical aerobic exercises include *walking* – which you can do at your own pace then increase to a more brisk, deliberate speed.

Stair climbing: Climb stairwells or use a stair-climbing machine. *Bicycling:* On the road or in the home or gym. *Jogging* burns a lot calories in a short amount of time. Start out slow and build up. Start by alternating walking with jogging. Don't increase mileage too quickly. *Swimming* puts less stress on joints and bones, and combines strength training, flexibility, and aerobic activity. *Dancing* is a great moderate-intensity activity and is lots of fun. Wear appropriate shoes and clothing. If you throw on a ragged T-shirt or sweats, it's not very inspiring for your workout. Start slowly. If you're sore or tired, give yourself extra recovery days. Remember that exercise, like happiness, is a journey, not a destination.

To get more health and weight-reduction benefits, add more time of aerobic physical activity. Try to move from 3 hours of moderate-level activities a week to five hours or more a week. If you're already doing 3 hours a week of aerobic physical activity, slowly add more time to your weekly routine. Strive to double your weekly activity time.

Add more effort. Instead of doing only moderate-level activities, replace some with vigorous aerobic activities that will make your heart beat even faster. Adding vigorous activities provides benefits in less activity time. In general, 15 minutes of vigorous activity provides the same benefits as 30 minutes of moderate activity. Have you been walking for 30 minutes five days a week? On two days, try jogging instead for 15 minutes each time. Keep on walking for 30 minutes on the other three days. Want stronger muscles? If you've been doing strengthening activities two days a week, try adding an extra day.

Target Heart Rate

The whole idea of aerobics is to get your heart rate high enough to benefit your cardiovascular system and to lose or maintain weight. So what's the correct Exercise Heart Rate for you, and how is it determined?

First, determine the intensity level at which you would like to exercise. If you've been a sedentary person, you may want to begin an exercise regimen at the 60% level and work up gradually to the 70% level. Athletes and highly fit individuals must work at the 85-95% level to receive the benefits of exercise.

Second, calculate the target heart rate (beats per minute). One common way of doing this is by using the ACSM Method. By this method you would subtract your age from 220, then multiply by the desired intensity level of the workout. This would give you your correct beats per minute. It's not practical to count heart beats for a whole minute, so divide the answer by 6 for a 10-second pulse count instead of a 60-second count. The 10-second pulse count is useful for checking whether the target heart rate is being achieved during the workout. One can easily check one's pulse at the wrist or side of the neck – counting the number of beats in 10 seconds.

For example, a 30-year-old wishing to exercise at 70% intensity, would use the following steps:

1. Maximum Heart Rate: 220 - 30 = 190

2. Target Heart Rate: 190 × .70 =133 (beats per minute)

3. Using 10-second (instead of 60-second) Pulse Count: 133 ÷ 6 = 22.

To work at the desired intensity level, this 30-year-old would strive for a target heart rate of 22.

Make your primary aerobic activity one that's measurable. The psychological reason for this is that you should be able to see progress if you expect to stay motivated. Remember that your stiff and sedentary body will be reluctant to change, just like a smoker's body will protest stopping smoking. Your job is to get that same body fit and slimmer so that it will protest when you *don't* exercise.

Strength Training

Strength-building exercises not only burn calories, they increase muscle mass. They also increase your calorie-burning metabolism – which can stay elevated for up to 48 hours after you've finished your exercise session. Strength training includes working with weights, doing calisthenics (sit-ups, push-ups, crunches, etc.), or any other resistance exercise. It targets specific body parts, making your muscles work against extra weight. Over time, the muscles become bigger to meet this demand. It can mean stronger bones, tendons, and ligaments; firmer, toned muscles; and a better sense of your body.

Eventually you can build up to 8 to 10 exercises per session that involve the major muscle groups. Do 8-12 repetitions of each exercise at least twice a week, with at least 1 day between activity sessions to allow muscles to recover. You can start with simple equipment such as 2- to 15-pound hand weights. Or use resistance bands made of strong, flexible elastic – available at sporting-goods stores. These bands can help strengthen arm and leg muscles.

Flexibility Training

Essentially, flexibility is stretching. It's the nudging of your physical boundaries. Building flexibility keeps you limber by lengthening your muscles, tendons, and ligaments. It may also decrease your risk of injury, and help you recover faster from injuries. It can help with improved freedom of movement, better posture, and increased physical and mental relaxation. After your warmup and after you finish your activity, stretch to help your muscles recover from what you've just done. Start slowly with each stretch and take deep breaths. Try to hold the stretch for 10 to 30 seconds. Don't bounce. If you feel any pain, it may be a sign you're doing too much. A few stretches after you've been sitting or standing for a while also can help you feel more energized. Some quick stretches you can try include: hamstring stretch, groin stretch, triceps stretch, hip stretch, thigh stretch, and upper arm and chest stretch. Check the Internet for free and low-cost videos of these stretches.

An example of a flexibility/yoga exercise would be the *Upper Body Twist* – which you can do standing or sitting. If sitting, sit tall, with your feet flat on the floor and shoulder-width apart. Place your hands behind your head with elbows pointing out to the sides. Twist your body to one side so your shoulders are parallel to the side wall, or as far as you can turn. Your head should follow your trunk. Slowly switch to the other side. Repeat six to eight times on each side.

Gradually work up to where you're stretching for 10 minutes at least three days a week. Try to involve the major muscles of the arms, legs, and torso. Hold stretches for 10 to 30 seconds and aim for three to four repetitions of each stretch (with a slight pause between reps).

Yoga practice is the ultimate in flexibility training. You can take a Tai Chi or Yoga class or buy or rent training videos. Yoga is a system of exercises to promote mind and body control. For centuries, yoga has been prescribed as moving medicine for the immune system.

Yoga has been reported to lower stress hormones that compromise immunity, while stimulating the lymphatic system to purge toxins and bring fresh, nutrient-oxygenated blood to each organ to help ensure optimum functioning. It is universally accepted for six thousand years that Yoga is highly beneficial in controlling and reversing many diseases and it can help you get rid of excessive fat.

Yoga is a combination of a set of physical and breathing exercises coupled with meditation. Each set of exercises are meant to address certain problems in the body and most people practice only those which they need. This could be controlling of blood pressure, diabetes, depression, arthritis, asthma, digestion, and so on. For your purpose, you want to also apply it to your weight loss goal – controlling the appetite and between-meal cravings, increasing metabolic rate, and relieving the stress which is the key trigger to most overeating episodes. (See Chapter 7, *How to Control Stress.*)

Recreational and Physical Activity

Along with Aerobics, Strength, and Flexibility exercises, you'll also want to be involved in some kind of both recreational activity – 2-3 days per week, and general physical activity – almost daily.

There are numerous activities that can be worked into your day that do not involve going to the gym, or an aerobics class. For example, walking is a very beneficial exercise most anyone can do.

Do it with a friend, find a local trail. Park as far away from your destination as possible and walk. If you live in town, walk to do your errands. Take a walk during your lunch break. Walk your dog, walk the beach, walk the mall, walk to errands. Take the stairs whenever you can. Avoid elevators and escalators. If you work on the 20th floor, take the elevator to the 15th floor and walk the last five flights.

Take up a sport. Call your local parks and recreation department and find out about local softball, basketball, racket sports, soccer, etc. Jump Rope. Play Games. In-line skate, swim, bicycle, tap dance, belly dance, jazz, social and Ballroom dance. Take advantage of classes being offered in your community and have a great time while you're at it.

Try some of these outdoor activities: Gardening is strenuous work. Get outside and play in the dirt. Use a hand mower on the lawn instead of a riding mower. Go hiking, canoeing, sailing, surfing. Wash and wax your car. Clean your house. Vacuuming, mopping and dusting can be a good workout. Do simple stretching and calisthenics exercises at your desk. Do anything that gets you up and moving, and most important, have fun. Think of it this way: You get leaner and leaner every time you move your body.

Pick an activity you like and one that fits into your life. Find the time that works best for you. Be active with friends and family. Having a support network can help you keep up with your program. There are many ways to build the right amount of activity into your life. Every little bit adds up and doing something is better than doing nothing. Here are two examples for adding more activity. You can do more by being active longer each time. Walking for 30 minutes, three times a week? Go longer – walk for 50 minutes, three times a week. You can do more, by being active more often. Are you biking lightly three days a week for 25 minutes each time? Increase the number of days you bike. Work up to riding six days a week for 25 minutes each time. If you have not been this active in the past, work your way up. In time, replace some moderate activities with vigorous activities that take more effort.

Mix and Match

You can do all moderate activities, all vigorous activities, or some of each. You should always start with moderate activities and then add vigorous activities little by little. To vary it, you can try 30 minutes of biking fast to and from your job three days a week. Then play doubles-tennis for 60 minutes one day. Then lift weights for two days. You've mixed vigorous aerobic activity (biking fast) with moderate aerobic activity (doubles-tennis) and activities for stronger muscles (weights). To add more effort, try some vigorous activities such as aerobic dance, fast Ballroom dance, jumping rope, martial arts (such as Karate), race walking, jogging, running, riding a bike on hills or riding faster, Soccer, swimming fast, Tennis (singles), etc.

You can choose moderate or vigorous activities, or a mix of both each week. You should do at least 3 hours each week of aerobic physical activity at a moderate level. Or you should do at least one hour and 15 minutes each week of aerobic physical activity at a vigorous level.

Pick an activity that's easy to fit into your life. Do at least 20 minutes of physical activity at a time. Choose aerobic activities that work for you. These make your heart beat faster and can make your heart, lungs, and blood vessels stronger and more fit. Also, do strengthening activities which make your muscles do more work than usual.

How many times a week you should be physically active is up to you, but it is better to spread your activity throughout the week and to be active at least three days a week. Do a little more each time. Once you feel comfortable, do it more often. Then you can trade activities at a moderate level for vigorous ones that take more effort. You can do moderate and vigorous activities in the same week.

The Talk Test

This is a simple way to measure relative intensity. As a rule of thumb, if you're doing moderate-intensity activity you can talk, but not sing, during the activity. If you're doing vigorous-intensity activity, you will not be able to say more than a few words without pausing for a breath. Here are just a few moderate and vigorous aerobic activities. Do these for 20 minutes or more at a time.

Moderate-Intensity Activities

While performing the physical activity, if your breathing and heart rate is noticeably faster but you can still carry on a conversation – it's probably moderately intense. Examples include walking briskly (a 15-minute mile), light yard work (raking/bagging leaves or using a lawn mower), light snow shoveling, actively playing with children, biking at a casual pace. Ballroom and line dancing, biking on level ground or with few hills, canoeing, general gardening (raking, trimming shrubs), sports where you catch and throw (baseball, softball, volleyball), Tennis (doubles), hand cyclers – also called ergometers, walking briskly, water aerobics, etc.

You can replace some or all of your moderate activity with vigorous activity. With vigorous activities, you get similar weight reduction benefits in half the time it takes you with moderate ones. Physical activity is generally safe for everyone. People who are physically fit have less chance of injury than those who are not fit. The health benefits you gain from being active are far greater than the chances of getting hurt. Being inactive is definitely not good for your health or for losing weight.

Here are some things you can do to stay safe while you are active: If you haven't been active in a while, start slowly and build up. Learn about the types and amounts of activity that are right for you. Choose activities that are appropriate for your fitness level. Build up the time you spend before switching to activities that take more effort. Use the right safety gear and sports equipment. Choose a safe place to do your activity. See a health care provider if you have a health problem or question.

Vigorous-Intensity Activities

With these activities, you can only say a few words without stopping to catch your breath. These include aerobic dance, biking faster than 10 miles per hour, fast dancing, heavy gardening (digging, hoeing), hiking uphill, jumping rope, martial arts (such as Karate) race walking, jogging, running. Sports with a lot of running (basketball, hockey, soccer.), swimming fast or swimming laps, Tennis (singles). To maintain your weight: Work your way up to 150 minutes of moderate-intensity aerobic activity, 75 minutes of vigorous-intensity aerobic activity, or an equivalent mix of the two each week. Strong scientific evidence shows that physical activity can help you maintain your weight over time. However, the exact amount of physical activity needed to do this is not clear since it varies greatly from person to person. It's possible that you may need to do more than the equivalent of 3 hours of moderate-intensity activity a week to maintain your weight.

Do the Math

Since 1 pound of fat = 3500 calories, losing 1 pound of excess weight per week means that 3500 calories of fat must be removed from storage and converted to energy per week. That's 3500 calories burned per week in excess of calories taken in, or 500 calories per day (3500 calories divided by 7 days). The way to achieve 2 pounds per week weight reduction is by consumption of 1000 fewer calories per day than are burned. This differential between calories eaten and calories burned is the only way to remove excess weight. (See the Physical Activity Chart in Appendix 4 and the Exercise Log in Appendix 5.)

Key Points and Principles to Remember from Chapter 4:

1. Commit to a physical exercise regimen that you can live with for life;

2. Plan your exercise routine in advance;

3. Keep a journal of your exercise session goals and achievements;

4. In general, exercise 20 to 60 minutes a day, 3 to 5 days a week;

5. Do moderate-intensity *Aerobic Exercises* at least 3 hours a week, or vigorous-intensity for 75 minutes a week;

6. Do *Strength Exercises* at least twice a week: 8-12 reps of 8-10 exercises;

7. Do *Flexibility Exercises* for 15 minutes at least 3 days a week – 3-4 repetitions of each stretch, holding each for 10-30 seconds;

8. Do *Recreational Activities* 2-3 days a week: swim, dance, bicycle, tennis;

9. Do some kind of *Physical Activity* almost daily for at least 20 minutes: walking, housecleaning, gardening, car washing;

10. Reward yourself for the steady progress that you're making. (See reward suggestions in Chapter 3.)

CHAPTER 5

HOW THE UNIVERSE WORKS"

The universe seems neither benign nor hostile, merely indifferent."
– Carl Sagan

Indifference, detachment and freedom are synonymous.

We now move our discussion from the body back to the mind. We go from the local gym to the universe as a whole, to gain some perspective and clues on how the mind works – or is supposed to work regarding life and mind/body management.

The experts tell us that the most effective and efficient way to be successful at something is – not to reinvent the wheel, but to copy that which is *already* successful. Simply find what works, then imitate it.

The Universal Success Formula

The universe as a whole is a wonderful success in that it supports and sustains *life, consciousness and happiness* – the three elements also essential to appetite-control power. If we dissect the universe to isolate the principal factor behind its success, we find that it's *centered* or *balanced*. The universe is the all-encompassing government, and being centered is its constitutional law, its central organizing principle. Centeredness then, is indicated for us, personally, because what works for the whole works for the part and vice versa.

That something is universal means it applies in every direction and on all levels and departments of life. We can find balance at work reducing tension and increasing efficiency everywhere, not only on the material, psychological, emotional and sensual levels but also morally, economically, politically, socially, ecologically, nutritionally, and so on.

To name just a few: The balance of power between national alliances relaxes political tension; the balance between church and state relaxes ideological tension; the balanced budget within a country, and the balance of trade between countries, reduces economic tension; the balance between plants and animals and their food and water reduce ecological tension; the stock and commercial markets are relaxed or comfortable when there is a balance between buyer and seller and supply and demand. We seek to balance our losses with profits, our liabilities with assets, our expenses with income. Justice in the court is based on balance between prosecution and defense. Our decision to buy a thing is not based on price alone or quality alone, but on the balance between them. In labor relations we strive to balance the needs of both employees and employers. In politics, balance is maintained by the pushing and pulling activities of the Democrats and Republicans, the liberals and conservatives. The success of a constitutional government is based on maintaining balance between the executive, legislative and judicial branches, and so on, indefinitely. Thus, the world is an orderly, harmonious structure with balance or centeredness the central organizing and controlling principle, the direction toward which all things move for optimal functioning (goal achievement).

This law of balance not only orders the direction of all activity, but orders the form and function of everything that exists as well. It determines a thing's structure and its use. For example, the front half of a sheet of paper is balanced by its back half, and it's because of this balanced form that it can now be used to write on. The balance between the inside and outside halves of a tea cup allow it to function as a container. This balanced nature of all things is such an obvious fact of existence that we commonly fail to notice it. All things must have two opposite sides. Every inner is balanced by an outer; every front must have a back; every up, a down. There can't be a good without a bad, a right without a wrong, a pleasure without a pain. Balance is what makes a thing whole and complete and can be expressed in the simple mathematical equation: one-half plus one-half equals a whole. Three parts in one.

How does this "success formula" relate to us personally? What are the three interrelated parts that constitute us? In other words, who are we? The first part of us is *life*. We are alive. The second part of us is *conscious*. We're conscious of being alive. And the third part is the effect or outcome of the first two – which is *happiness*. Awareness that we are alive *results* in happiness. And the more aware of life we are, the happier we are. Happiness is the fulfillment of the equation, the fulfillment of conscious living. These are the three interrelated parts that form our true self, our higher, appetite-controlled self. Happiness is the purpose of life just as a container is the purpose of a cup. Happiness is the fruit of the union, the product of the marriage of Life and Consciousness.

Consciousness "knew" Life and conceived a child whose name was Happiness or Love. Happiness is of the heart, soul or *center*. It is the "spiritual" part of us, the invisible, appetite-controlling part of us – for if you have this real love or happiness, there's no need or desire to under eat, overeat, over drink, over work – anything negative or unhealthy whatsoever.

The difference, then, between emotional happiness and spiritual happiness is that the emotional is of the lower, personal self; while spiritual or *real* happiness is of the higher, *im*personal self. Emotional happiness is self-centered, while spiritual, consciousness-of-life happiness, is neutrally or universally centered.

Wholeness is the integration of all three parts. We can't be conscious of life and remain unhappy, and we can't be happy while unconscious of life. When holistically centered this way, we are our true selves, our fully empowered selves; in full and effortless control of our appetites. And, again, the way to be more conscious is to be more detached from whatever you're conscious of – especially that of eating.

Waking Up

The purpose of being centered is to awaken consciousness. That was its purpose in the beginning and that remains its purpose. To illustrate, let's turn the evolutionary clock back to our embryonic stage. In the beginning, life existed, and we were it. We were alive but not yet aware of it – as many of us are right now. We were as if in a state of deep sleep where all of our vital functions continued to operate and develop without conscious involvement. The time would come when we would awaken to the fact of life's existence, but first, certain conditions would have to mature or evolve. We were like a seed which inherently contained the complete blueprint of what it would become, but in order to germinate and bloom to that potential, we must first be exposed to the right mixture of nourishing soil, sun and water.

Our goal and creative task, then, as a budding young organism would be to somehow evolve those conditions which would allow our consciousness to awaken. The main problem, or rather, the *catch* to be overcome in accomplishing this goal will have to do with a certain law of relativity or relationship. This law says that personal knowledge is a relative thing – meaning that *we can't know anything unless in relation or contrast with its opposite.* The "opposite" provides the contrast necessary to make a thing stand out and be noticed. Opposites act like mirrors that reveal each others' presence. For example, we wouldn't notice pleasure without pain. If it weren't for intermittent pain we wouldn't recognize or appreciate pleasure. Pain is the very thing that makes pleasure so pleasing. Pain, then, not only opposes pleasure, but complements it as well. They are two sides of the same coin, two sides of the same mind.

Wherever there is sameness we fail to notice; we can't discriminate. A polar bear lying in the snow is virtually invisible. We don't notice the hair style of a person we see everyday until it's been changed. We don't notice the homes on our own street because the sameness of the scene has dulled our awareness. It's only when a house has been re-painted or removed that we realize it had ever existed. It is *contrast* that stimulates awareness. Similarly, we wouldn't know day as day unless it alternated with night. We wouldn't know cold as cold unless there was such a thing as hot to compare it with, and so on with all pairs of opposites – including life and death. And there was our problem – that in order to *know* life, we'd have to *know* death. What to do? It seems illogical, contradictory, paradoxical!

When death is reached, it would seem too late to experience life because then we're dead – that is, unless we somehow *came to life at the point of death* – which seems to be exactly what we did. There is a split moment during the life to death transition when this law of relationship is fulfilled and an awakening of consciousness occurs. It is that split second when life is leaving but has not yet left, and when death is approaching but has not yet arrived. In between them is a minute crossover point. A point of transcendence. A paradoxical moment when there is *neither* life nor death, and at the exact same time there are *both* life and death. They overlap or superimpose each other so that, in effect, each contains the character of the other at the same time. It's like a composite or trick photograph that's produced by overlapping different negatives. Or it's like a person straddling the border line between two states, whereby he's at the same time in *both* states and in *neither* state. He's centered or poised between them.

It's a very subtle moment, one of infinitesimal duration, like the moment between the in-breath and out-breath. Or like the moment when a ball thrown into the air is no longer rising but has not yet begun to fall. It is simultaneously *not* rising and *not* falling, and at the same time it *is* rising and *is* falling. It's balanced in the middle, relaxed between the "up" and the "down."

The ball has attained to a state of equilibrium or relaxation. The centrifugal force which threw the ball up is now equal to the gravitational force which would bring it down. The ball has now, in effect, transcended time and space. It's neither in the past nor in the future. It is neither moving nor still. It is neither up nor down. It is in this vacuum, this void, this state of *centered relaxation* that an awakening of consciousness occurs.

The problem to overcome, then, was that *real* death was not very practical to use as an opposite or mirror through which to see we were alive. The solution became this: *create the illusion or effect of death.* This could be accomplished by creating a universe with a system of equilibrium that exactly duplicates that state of centered relaxation – *but on an ongoing, continuous basis instead of for just a split-second*. In other words, we would continuously and indefinitely be alive, conscious, blissful – and of course, lean.

Constructing a Centered Universe

In the beginning, we didn't have a "physical" body, at least not one as heavy and coarse as we have now. At that time we consisted of a fine ethereal substance of incredible malleability. Gold, for instance, is so ductile that an ounce of it can be drawn into a strand of wire miles long. But the essential substance of our being is so exquisitely fine, that a dot less than the size of the period at the end of this sentence was drawn into a single, unbroken line that filled up all space in the entire universe – like water fills all the nooks and crannies of the ocean.

When we were just a dot beginning to expand out of our self to begin construction of a relative universe, we quickly realized that we could conserve energy by moving in the form of an up and down wavelike pattern instead of in a straight line. We expanded in one direction then rested an equivalent period in the opposite direction. We expanded and relaxed, expanded and relaxed. The opposites of "movement" and "relaxation" perfectly complemented each other. But the more marvelous thing about this strategy was that we expanded even during the relaxation part of the cycle and relaxed during the expansion part. It wasn't that we moved and *then* rested, we moved and rested simultaneously. We rested *while* moving and moved *while* resting. The gravity of the "down" movement built up so much momentum, like a speeding roller coaster, that instead of stopping at the bottom, it just continued up to the peak of the next cycle where gravity pulled it down again to repeat the process infinitely. The centrifugal force of the "up" movement perfectly balanced the gravitational force of the "down" rest. We vibrated forward in the same way that a fish wiggles forward. We were a perpetual-motion machine – a wonderfully efficient system of simultaneous movement and relaxation that allowed us to fill up the entire universe without effort or drain of energy.

For an indeterminate period afterward, we just moved about in a seemingly chaotic manner, in, around, and through our self like dough in a gigantic, slow-motion mixing machine – until all of a sudden we formed our self into a state of perfect equilibrium in which we became like the "zero" point at the center of a balance scale, where all the influences on our left became equal to all those on our right "balancing out" the effects of each other in the process. We took up the whole universe yet it was like we weren't there at all. Our weight balanced itself right out. We were so equally balanced, so equally opposed, so equally distributed, that we became, in effect, totally invisible, totally relaxed. Every "this" canceled every "that." A surplus here balanced a shortage there; an action here caused a reaction there. Every cause produced an effect and every effect had a cause. Every giving received and every taking diminished. It was one unified, balanced, interconnected, interrelated, harmonious whole. And at the center of it all, at the heart of it all, poised among all opposing influences, in a state of perfect relaxation and freedom, was where we were. At that moment, consciousness dawned on us. We awoke!

For a while, we just laid there, as when we sometimes awaken from a deep sleep and don't quite realize it immediately, but just stare out blankly for a few seconds before knowing, "Oh, I'm awake." We looked out with eyes of awareness now open and realized that we were alive, that we were living, that life was happening and it was happening through us. We were the medium of life and simultaneously, a witness to it as well. Self-conscious. How awesome is that? And since we were all there was, our perception was all pervasive and all knowing. We were as if made of the purest crystal, seeming not to be there at all, yet present everywhere. We were at once on the outside looking in, and on the inside looking out; at once the subject and the object; at once the beginning and the end.

For a sense of this experience, imagine yourself standing on a vast grassy plain. All around you for as far as the eye can see, there is only level plush grass meeting a wide open, cloudless blue sky at a huge circular horizon. It's like being in the top half of great blue bubble. Now, while remaining alert and fearless, allow the entire ground you're standing on to completely disappear so that the bottom half of the blue bubble meets the top half, with you just floating in the middle of a peaceful sea of blue. The sky is no longer just up, but is now everywhere; it's all around you. You are now *in* the sky.

Now, again, while remaining alert and fearless, allow your entire physical, personal body to disappear so that all that remains is pure impersonal awareness. The final umbilical cord has been severed. There are no more boundaries; no more separations or distinctions. You are no longer *in* the sky, now you *are* the sky. There is no difference between you and the sky. You've become one with it, one with all that exists. To the knowledge that you were alive, you could only respond with a bliss whose glow lovingly pervaded the entire universe. "Oh, the wonder and sweetness of it. The utter gloriousness of it. I am a living thing. Something is, and I am that! It's like a great mirror has folded in two to reveal myself, to know myself, to find myself, to control myself."

Realizing Your Potential

Notice now that of the three elements comprising the Universal Success Formula, only consciousness is controllable. Life is fixed, and happiness is tied to consciousness – the more aware you are, the more happy; the less aware, the less happy. Consciousness, then, is the only element that's controllable, and detachment is the means by which to control it.

Now people come in various degrees of consciousness. Some of us just barely know we're alive, and a handful of us are fully enlightened. But the masses of us are conscious to only about ten-percent of our potential. This means that only ten-percent of our self has been realized. We are only ten-percent as alive, happy, and personally effective as we could be at any given moment. The other ninety-percent remains untapped potential.

The subconscious ninety-percent contains all the intelligence that makes up our total organism. It contains the brilliant guidance system that led us, and continues to lead us, from darkness to consciousness. It is the organism that pumps our blood, digests our food, breathes our oxygen, heals our wounds, adjusts hormones and metabolism, etc. – even as we sleep. It's on constant alert twenty-four hours a day, never ceasing to serve us. It is an organism of exquisite perfection whose sole purpose is our beneficence. It is infinite love, intelligence and power, all rolled into one.

The subconscious contains all the knowledge of the universe from the beginning to the end. This is too much knowledge for the human brain to handle all at once. It would be as blinding as staring at the sun. We can only access the subconscious in small bits, and only to the degree we are not affected by the knowledge we receive. The more detached we are, the more truth we can handle, the more happiness, intelligence and power we can handle.

The goal of human evolution is a movement away from *personal* self-consciousness toward neutral self-consciousness – spiritual self-consciousness. It's a moving away from experiencing life from a narrow, personal perspective, to a more holistic, universal perspective. It's viewing ourselves both as an integral part of the situation or relationship we're in as well as an outsider looking in. That's what being centered is. Objective and subjective at the same time. All inclusive. This is the state where anything that is not the real you – like your ECH, is totally demolished, immolated in the fire of truth.

We make a situation what it is as it makes us what we are, simultaneously. We are not separate from the situation (the universe) but are directly integrated with it, hard-wired into it. We are never innocent bystanders in any situation. Our presence alters it in some way, and that alteration spreads like ripples on the surface of a pond. Homicide detectives say there can be no such thing as a perfect crime because the perpetrator *must* always leave something of his presence at the scene, however minute. All he needs is equipment or perception sensitive enough to detect it.

Remember that we just created the *illusion* of being separate or different in order to provide the contrast necessary to become conscious. Our organism (universe) was and is perfect, but *artificially* became imperfect or imbalanced only for the purpose of providing the impetus or stimulation necessary to begin "material" creation or manifestation (for when you are perfect, you don't really *need* to do anything). Our tendency now is to heal, so to speak, to return to centered relaxation, wholeness, truth — only this time, not just as a living being, but as a fully conscious, happy, fulfilled and slimmer one as well.

It is of course only natural that in order to become *un*self-conscious, you have to first be *self*-conscious. A thing has to be known before it can be let go. Once you *know* something, you don't have to think about it any longer; you rise above it. Once a child learns to walk or ride a bike, he needn't give it another thought. It has become "natural" and the mechanical details of it can be forgotten. Likewise, in order to forget yourself there must first be a self to forget. You can't forget yourself until you find yourself, and you can't find yourself until you forget yourself. Only then can you be in natural control of yourself and your appetite. In other words, you had to be fat before you could get the idea of being lean, that there was such a thing and possibility as being and staying lean.

Centered relaxation (not thinking or desiring at all) resolves or transcends this paradox by returning you back to the center of balance, back to the "zero" point where both your lower, personal self and your higher, subconscious self simultaneously coexist. In this way you are, and you naturally express, your healthy, happy and powerful self to the fullest without being conscious of it in the slightest.

Key Points and Principles to Remember from Chapter 5:

1. *Balance* is the central organizing and controlling principle of everything in the universe — including what and how you think, feel and eat;

2. Balance awakens consciousness of whatever you're thinking, feeling and eating;

3. Balance nullifies all negative feelings, habits and conditions;

4. Self-control is the result of happiness, which is the result of increased consciousness, which is the result of increased detachment from thoughts, feelings and food;

5. Whatever you want to be, do or have in life is already contained in your subconscious mind and is yours for the detached asking.

CHAPTER 6

HOW TO BE CENTERED

"Being Centered is the goal; detachment is the way."

To be centered is to be physically relaxed, emotionally calm, mentally focused and consciously above it all. Control of the emotions is so essential to quality of life in general and to appetite-control in particular, that four chapters are devoted to it. This chapter emphasizes how emotions affect your clarity and power; the next, how to control pain, pleasure and stress; Chapter 9, on Meditation shows you how to cultivate being centeree centered in a concentrated way; and Chapter 10 shows how being centered can exist only in the present moment.

How clearly you see a thing depends on how calmly centered you are. When centered, you know what you're doing, and only do what you know. Things then fall into place for you without stress or strain, and your goals are achieved as a matter of course. But when you're disturbed or excited about something painful *or* pleasurable, the opposite becomes the case – you lose yourself. You lose your relaxation and objectivity and *think* you know what you're doing rather than *know* you know. Self-control then becomes an effort and a struggle. Things don't go as planned and you experience frustration and disappointment as a result.

The Vicious Circle

Let's look at, not only how emotional stress affects your ability to see clearly, but also how it sets off a chain reaction process by which the problem is perpetuated indefinitely, and without your even being aware of it. Have you ever been so sure of something only to find you were totally wrong about it? Wasn't it bewildering? Maybe it was a personal or business decision or idea, or the choosing of a financial investment or marriage partner; you had considered everything so carefully. You had no doubt it was right, that it would work – then it crashed and you wondered what went wrong.

This is what happened: Instead of basing your decision on matters relating to the issue in and of itself, you became excitedly or tensely involved in it. Such involvement affected your ability to remain impartial or centered. Instead of seeing all sides of the situation dispassionately in order to make a fair judgment – you influenced it. You took it *personally* instead of neutrally. Your "personal" involvement contaminated the decision-making process. Your decision wasn't based on fact, but on the influential sway of your own personality. You colored the decision. You interfered with it. You unconsciously manipulated it to coincide with how you perhaps would've *liked* it to be, or how you believed it should, would or could be. In other words, the decision was *personally biased*, causing the outcome to be inevitably different than the way you envisioned it – different meaning negative, and negative meaning stress. The problem is perpetuated when we carry residual tension from past situations to the present, insuring it too will result negatively.

On a short-term basis, it's like a cartoon character upset over a flat tire and reacting by kicking it and stubbing his toe. Then in angry reaction he punches the fender and fractures his hand, then begins to scream obscenities, is arrested for disorderly conduct and put in a straightjacket. Or more commonly, it's like resentment over a poor Mah Jong play, and carrying that resentment over to negatively affect the next play, and the next, until your whole game is off, which would throw your whole day off. And if we extrapolate this cause and effect cycle, your whole week would be off, your whole month would be off and your whole life would be off.

Other examples would be fear of dogs because of being bitten as a child; fear of starting a new business venture because of a past failure; fear of closeness or openness in a relationship because of a past hurt; fear of committing to a new recovery method because of past disappointments, and so on. Thus are we involved in a three-way, chain reaction process where one, being stressed causes us to not see clearly what we're doing; two, not seeing clearly brings about a negative or undesired outcome; and three, the undesired outcome produces stress, which makes us not see clearly what we're doing all over again.

In a circle or cycle there's no difference between the beginning and the end; they are the same point. The way it works physically is the way it works mentally and emotionally. Whenever you enter the moment tensely, you set events into motion which will bring about tension in the end. If you're in error going in, you'll be frustrated coming out; if correct going in, you'll be satisfied coming out. What goes, comes; what gives, gets. The end is always a mirror reflection of the beginning. The very state of mind or body you're in right now is the one you'll return to when all is said and done. Your future body and eating behavior is nothing more than a projection of your present state of mind.

This is the basic principle, by the way, of how some fortune-tellers "read" whether upcoming circumstances will be favorable for you. To the degree you appear calm and composed, you could expect a positive outcome, but to the degree you appear conflicted or nervous, the opposite is indicated. – Things will probably not go well, so you'd be advised to not make any important personal or business decisions at that time.

The Right Attitude

The remedy becomes this: Change the beginning. Change the present. Willingness to change is the first step on the road to relaxation and disorder-control. "If nothing changes, nothing changes." And the thing to change is this: Enter each moment the way you want to come out of each moment – happy, content and free, regardless of what happened a second ago or twenty-years ago. This is the essence of the law of detachment.

Think of life as constantly cyclical, or as an infinite series of circles. Each circle is a new present-moment of unlimited possibilities; one you've never experienced before nor ever will again. You begin each present-moment cycle *knowing* and *expecting* that it will return full circle with the exact fruit with which it was germinated. Negative returns negative, positive returns positive.

Overcoming your food issue is a process of changing your attitude from the self-centered way you habitually perceive it and live in general. Life is not all about you, personally. It never was and never will be. It's also not happening *to* you; it's just happening. Period. That rude clerk wasn't insensitive to you, *personally*; he just happened to be in that state of mind, and you just happened to be handy. And that half glass of water isn't about optimism or pessimism; it's just a half glass of water. The personal view is an unreal, powerless *opinion* or *concept;* while the neutral, detached, universal view is a *fact.* Intelligence is not what you "think;" it's the relaxed, impersonal, objective, matter-of-fact way you look at things. It is this matter-of-fact viewpoint that allows you to see your eating disorder with such extraordinary clarity that fear, doubt and uncertainty are naturally eliminated, and all of your actions and responses become perfectly appropriate, effortless and effective.

Being detachedly centered, is nothing more than common sense, and although not so common, it's your natural and original state of being. It's who and what you really are. It's the way you were before you allowed the pressures and influences of the world to excite you off balance and out of control. Becoming centered is to regain that lost balance, and along with it, your lost beauty, dignity, joy, power and freedom.

Getting Control

Let's look at how taking life personally distorts your perception of reality, and in the process causes you to lose control of yourself; that is to say, causes your reactions to be controlled by people, places and things outside of you. Self-centeredness can be characterized as a form of paranoia in the sense, for example, that those who disagree with us, we tend to feel disagree with us *personally,* so we become upset or resentful. Conversely, we're inclined to feel that those who agree with us, agree with us *personally* – so we get a swelled head instead. Disagreement frazzles us; affirmation flatters us. One drags us down, the other lifts us up.

Self-centeredness causes music to affect us similarly. We tend to take it personally or to identify with it so that depending on the arrangement and tempo, it can sentimentally sink us into melancholy or stir us to cheeriness and optimism. It's due to this emotional swaying power of music that most commercial media are produced in the form of musical jingles. The "catchy" tunes influence our feelings and effectively hypnotize us into accepting or sympathizing with whatever product, person or idea is being sold. We act primarily according to how we *feel.* If our feelings can be externally controlled, then our actions and what we buy or believe can be externally controlled – and then we fully believe that it was our own decision.

Hypnosis is a simple two-step procedure of first capturing the subject's total attention, then planting a suggestion – which is then likely to be accepted. For example, if you were asked to concentrate on *not* thinking of an elephant, you'd *have* to think of an elephant in order to process that request. So, in effect, your thinking was "controlled" by that person. Another example of hypnosis would be that of a tourist in Manhattan staring up at the top of a skyscraper, and passers by seeing him look up, stop to look up too. Soon there is a crowd of people looking up. It's almost irresistible to *not* look up. That's the power of suggestion.

Through the medium of television, our attention is gained through the excitement or stimulation of the senses (sensationalism). Through the sense of sight, our attention is captured by rapid-fire scenes of beautiful young people frolicking on the beach. And through the sense of hearing our attention is held by the musical jingles and loud, fast-talking salespeople or cartoon characters. Without such sophisticated entrancement techniques we'd be more likely to see the product as it *really* is, rather than as we are being led to *imagine* or *believe* it is. We would see that the product's "image" and the actual product have little in common – that there's nothing really romantic or exciting about a soft drink, for instance, that may consist of nothing more than gas, chemicals and impure tap water.

Such is the way taking life personally, negatively effects your life – by altering your perception of reality, and by controlling your reactions so that you're not really your own person, but a semi-conscious, easily suggestible victim of circumstances. It's no wonder you think there's something wrong with yourself or your body. The only thing wrong with you is your wrong response to the world.. You need to trust yourself more, and the world less. The world is just doing its own thing and so should you. Remember the perception-is-everything principle, don't allow it deceive you. Just be more centered, more discriminating so you

you're able to see through life. Get a life of your own. Be independent of the world as well as a part of it. Be a leader of our own life; not a follower. Stop thinking you need this food issue. It's okay to not have it.

Getting Indifferent

Taking life personally is seeing things one-sidedly and distortedly. We're stressed because we don't see the whole picture, and we don't because we're personally biased. The relaxed, centered point of view, on the other hand, works in the opposite. It relates to clarity of perception and tranquillity of mind. Being centered is seeing both sides of a situation with equal passion – like the pros and cons of a debate, for instance. Clarity is seeing a thing in its wholeness and completeness. Tranquillity means not being disturbed or excited by one side any more than the other. You're composed because you see the *whole* situation, and you see the whole situation because, as far as your higher consciousness is concerned, they're the same.

Being centered is mentally balancing yourself between the two sides of any issue. It's being established in a position or attitude of neutrality with respect to all that you see, hear, think, feel and do, whether it's external or internal, painful or pleasurable. To be centered is like being a juror at a trial where fairness and justice depend on your ability to remain impartial. The prosecution is biased toward the state; the defense is biased toward the defendant. It's only for you, the witnessing, impartial juror, to remain detached. In order to make a right and fair judgment, you have to consider the evidence presented by both sides with complete equanimity.

Life itself is like a court trial in that getting to the truth is the whole object of it. It's to view the evidence of it, determine the facts of it, get to the heart of it. The prosecution and defense are like negative and positive thoughts and feelings. We are the impartial observers, the neutral witnesses to these thoughts and feelings. The prosecuting thought says, "You're wrong." The defending thought says, "No, you're right." One says, "Eat this," the other, "No, eat that." Which shall you believe and follow? You cannot believe either because both are biased opinions so are irrelevant, immaterial and incompetent.

Through maintaining a centered perspective, you rise above such internal conflict and allow the truth of a thing to become revealed and the way to go to become obvious. Whenever you have conflicted feelings about something, it's because you're looking at it one-sidedly. You are somehow being partial or prejudiced.

If you're having mixed feelings over whether to eat that hot fudge sundae, for example, it's because your feelings want it but the mental doesn't think you should. There's a division, split or conflict, which indicates the wrong time or thing to eat at that time – not because the mind is superior in judgment to the heart, or vice versa, but because there's an imbalance operating, and whenever there's imbalance, there'll be error – and the consequent regret.

Here the heart says "Yes, a hot fudge sundae would be really good," but the mind says, "No, no. Don't do it. Think of the fat and calories. Think of how many miles you'll have to run to pay for it. Think of what a new wardrobe of large-size clothing would cost!" But deep down in the subconscious the choice has *already* been made. Sure, you'll rationalize it, intellectualize it, consider it from every possible angle, but we both know that sundae is going to prevail. It's like subjecting the sundae to a kangaroo court where it's given a "fair" trial before it's eaten.

Clarity comes from seeing a situation in its *wholeness,* which comes from being centered in the middle of it. Seeing a thing wholly and completely is like the superior view the manager of a company has over his subordinates in the various departments. The manager of a hotel, for instance, is aware of *all* the various functions of a hotel's operation and how they are interrelated. The hotel is an organization with the manager centered among all functions. The front desk, housekeeping, sales, maintenance, accounting, and food and beverage departments, are all on the periphery. Each department is biased, so to speak; each seeing only its own narrow, limited *part* of the operation and virtually blind to the other parts, while the manager has a *view of the whole.*

Being centered between opposite poles is like the lifeguard who, standing still (relaxed) at the center of the beach – the point of maximum visibility, is more effective than one who moves (emotes) back and forth from one extreme end of the beach to the other. The "centered" lifeguard sees the whole beach at all times; the "biased" lifeguard sees only part of the beach at a time, while leaving the opposite part always unattended. The mind that's still sees clearly; the mind that moves sees distortedly.

The mind works like binoculars or a camera: The more still it's held, the clearer the view or sharper the image. In another sense, the mind works like a chimney and damper. When the damper (the viewpoint) is straight up and down (centered), the smoke (what you see and hear) can flow without being altered. But to the degree the damper is leaning to the left or to the right (being partial or prejudiced), it blocks the free passage of smoke. And while it's blocking it, it's also distorting it. Instead of the smoke passing directly and immediately out, it must now twist and contort itself around the damper, so the smoke now exiting the chimney is totally different (false) than the smoke that entered.

The Mind is Merely a Medium

All that you perceive must pass through the mind in order to be understood. The mind, like the chimney and damper, functions as a conduit through which information may be processed. The higher, subconscious mind, of itself, is not designed to *do* anything; it is only a *medium* of expression or passage. Its job is to be *the master reference point* of perception and action. It's job is to remain as centered as possible, as "straight up and down" as possible. That's its most unobtrusive, unaffected position. It is then, in effect, not there at all, as when air currents turn a hanging mobile sideways so that it "appears" to have disappeared. As far as the smoke is then concerned, there is no damper. The smoke can now pass without interference and without its nature or character altered in the process.

You want free will. You want high-fidelity perception. You don't want what you see and hear to be affected on the way to our understanding. You want to get exactly what you we see, and see exactly what you're getting. When the letter carrier delivers your mail, he doesn't open it to correct the grammar or rewrite it to make it sound better. He delivers it *as is.*

Getting Unaffected

Being centered is being relaxed, content, poised, detached, self-controlled, unaffected. To illustrate, think of yourself as a child's seesaw – just a straight board. When you're a centered seesaw, you're unaffected by the "ups" and "downs" of your life, because when a part of you goes up, the opposite part of you goes down an equal degree, so that your straightness or integrity is not violated; that is, you don't get "all bent out of shape." The weight or influence on one end cancels that on the opposite end, for a net effect on you of *zero.* And what's true physically, is true mentally and emotionally. When centered, the positive part of you cancels the negative part of you; what's pleasurable cancels what's painful, and so on with all pairs of opposites. As far as you, the unaffected seesaw are concerned, there is no good or bad, right or wrong, pain or pleasure. Such things are relative and exist only to the degree you choose to sit on that particular extreme.

Being unaffected is like being in the position of a broker or middleman whose profit comes from the transaction itself, so is indifferent to the personalities of the buyers and sellers involved. It makes no difference if Mr. Pain is the buyer and Mr. Pleasure is the seller, or vice versa – Mr. Middleman still gets paid. But on the other hand, if Mr. Middleman only desires Mr. Pleasure and avoids Mr. Pain, then the situation would be imbalanced. No sale could take place, and Mr. Middleman *would* be affected. Similarly, the owner of a pari-mutual race track is unaffected by the amounts won or lost by virtue of his middleman position. Every dollar won is balanced by a dollar lost. After deducting expenses and his percentage, the proceeds from the losers are equally divided among the winners. The negative effect of the winning tickets is canceled out by the positive effect of the losing tickets. The owner remains calm and content. He's indifferent to whether you win or lose; it's all the same to him. His only concern is that you play the game. For the middleman, the centered and relaxed man, there is no winning or losing; there is only the joy and profit of the transaction. Freedom from affectation and wrong eating then, involves cultivating an equal appreciation for both winning and losing, for both pain and pleasure.

Life is such that sometimes you win, sometimes lose. Sometimes there's pleasure, sometimes pain. Sometimes you're the buyer, sometimes the seller. They are two equal and inseparable sides of the same coin, the same mind; so being affected by one side more than the other is incompatible with reality. As life includes both, your embrace and acceptance should include both, for you *are* life. This is living on *life's* terms not on personally-biased, self-centered terms.

You, the higher you, is not designed to have even a *preference* for winning, for pleasure, for sunshine. Emotional preferences, like emotional desire, are the very cause of the anxiety and stress that block happiness and self-control. Simply point your nose toward your intention and assume you've already attained it. Then go about your business creatively instead of emotionally. Know your role, task or purpose at any given moment and involve yourself in it from the position of your higher, centered self. If it turns out negative, you won't be disturbed. If it turns out positive, you don't get excited – for the uncontrolled excitement of success will prevent your maintaining or repeating it.

Holding a personal preference is holding a personal *pressure*, and is just as erroneous and harmful as being externally pressured. To be pressured is to be tilted off balance, which would tend to bring the opposite of what you want – as in the seesaw illustration. Feeling pressure at school, for example, would disturb your concentration. Pressure from a friend or family member would estrange your relationship. Pressure at work would stifle your creativity. Pressure to produce or perform would inhibit performance. Pressure to conform would cause you to rebel. Pressure to lose weight would cause you to gain more weight. Pressure to stop a bad habit would strengthen its grip on you. Financial pressure would block your resourcefulness, and so on. The detached attitude neutralizes pressure, so you function more fully, efficiently, effectively, spontaneously, naturally and effortlessly.

Those who claim to operate better under pressure are really subconsciously addicted to it. The person who *needs* pressure in order to function is wrongly motivated. The rightly motivated person works first for the work itself, for the action itself. Success follows as a natural side effect. But the wrongly motivated person has it backwards: He works for the side effect first – the money (or body) first, for example. He has a problem, for once he's financially comfortable, there's no longer any "real" reason to be productive, so he must create artificial pressure through the emotional, endless pursuit of more and more expensive toys, entertainments and diversions. He spins in a circle like a mouse on a spending-to-earn, earning-to-spend treadmill. Once he arrives at each new plateau of so-called success, he crashes into the reality of the unfulfillment and emptiness of it. He finds higher and higher mountains to climb only to end up where he began –

hungry and discontent. Only if he lives long enough does he come to realize that the top is not where "it" is at; where it's at is in the journey. It's en route. It's in the infinite action – as we discussed earlier. It's always in the exact spot where one happens to be standing at any given moment. The top of the self-control mountain is not a place; it's a state of mind right here and now.

Raising Your Emotional Thermostat

Now being centered along with its increased clarity, joy and power, does not necessarily come all at once, but only to the degree you can handle it. Obviously, if you become overly excited you're not centered any longer. That's the catch. Detachment allows awareness to increase, but as soon as it does, excitement about it immediately blocks its continuance. So you move one step forward, one step backward, either not growing at all or growing at the pace of a snail. This up and down relaxation/excitement cycle works like a thermostat control: clarity, joy and power rise to the point of excitement – then shut off. Your task becomes raising the excitement point higher and higher so that self-control can rise correspondingly. In other words, you want to become less and less excited about more and more things. Wisdom and power, are nothing more than the ability to either enjoy or suffer without making an emotional issue of it. Feelings are just feelings, and the more relaxed and detached you are, the more above and in control of all feelings.

Stress itself is a neutral energy but becomes negative when you get carried away by it, and becomes positive when kept under control, that is, kept neutral. Being controlled is not being "cold" as commonly misinterpreted. On the contrary, you not only feel the entire spectrum of human emotion, you feel it even *more* vividly, *more* passionately – but you're not excited or disturbed by it. Nothing in life should surprise you because there is simply no end to its novelty to the degree you venture from your self-imposed comfort zone.

Balance controls physical, mental, emotional and sensual energy so you can operate, grow and act more effectively and efficiently. Physical balance, such as pacing yourself during physical activity, controls and conserves that energy. Mental balance or stillness conserves psychic energy so you can think better. The nature of the body is to move, but the nature of the mind is to be still. If the body isn't exercised, its muscles atrophy; if the mind isn't stilled, intelligence and power atrophy. Emotional centeredness is how you control painful or pleasurable feelings so you don't get carried away by either. And sensual centeredness is what allows you to be more discriminating as to the quality, quantity and character of all you see, hear, taste, touch and smell – making it virtually impossible to eat the wrong thing or eat if for the wrong reason.

Getting Real

When centered, you're living in reality or *truth* – truth being defined here as that which exists *before* you personalize it, conceptualize it or emotionalize it. Now the only difference between being emotional and being relaxedly and detachedly centered is that in the one case, you're *out* of control, and in the other, *in* control. The emotional person is scattered; the centered person is collected. The emotional person is possessed by the world; the centered is self-possessed. The emotional can be excited or depressed by anything, while the centered person isn't excited or depressed by anything. The emotional person is a slave – for whatever inflates or depresses her, owns her. The centered person is free; the emotional person is disconnected from her source and center so is easily taken over – especially by food. The relaxed, centered person is connected to her center so is clear and confident as to why and when to eat and when to stop. Food is no more an issue in her life than is walking and talking. She eats when hungry and stops when the hunger has passed. She's not *doing* control; she's *being* control. Self-controlled is who she naturally is. It's not something that has to be thought about.

The word "excite" means to *move away*. To relax means to loosen back, to be restored to a previous condition. When you're relaxing, you're detaching back to your original state of effortless being – which is the state of centered relaxation. Living in detachment is living in your relaxed home, your ideal, your center of operations. Whenever you leave it, you feel discomfort; whenever you detach, you feel at ease. Stress or excitement is what pulls you away from that center, and detachment is what brings you back.

Being centered comes by degree, and to the degree you're centered in your being and outlook, you transcend being emotionally affected or disordered by anything – including food. On a lower level, you'd be unaffected by rain or sunshine; on a higher level, you'd remain unaffected even if that rain brought you financial disaster, for example. Your essential wise and good nature would not change, and you wouldn't leap from the roof of a building. Your spouse, children and dog might leave you. Your friends might be dismayed. The bank may take your home, and the Internal Revenue Service may padlock your business. You might even have to sleep in a public shelter and stand in soup lines, but none of this would uncontrollably distress you. You'd remain your calm and composed self. External conditions could not corrupt the real you, the beautiful you, the eternally poised and courageous you. – Of course, being so calm and clear you wouldn't come to such an extreme in the first place. You'd have anticipated the problem, or if not, you'd have had the creative power to make the necessary course corrections and bounce back.

The point is to become less and less affected by more and more things until you come to realize that nothing external can harm you; that it's only when you allow outside influences to get under your skin that your eating disorder begins; that even if you were at rock bottom you'd still be all right. You'd still survive, that you had always survived and that you always would; that there's indeed nothing to fear; that all that *appears* negative in life doesn't exist in objective reality, but is merely an illusion born of a self-centered outlook.

With higher degrees of unaffectedness, pain becomes less and less painful until you can't differentiate between it and pleasure. The dividing line between them diminishes until it disappears, and you're not sure whether you're supposed to laugh or cry. There are no more ups and downs. They become equal. The mountains lower and the valleys lift. Now there's only one you, not two. You've risen above all superficial distinctions of pain and pleasure, failure and success. Now there remains only joy, peace and contentment. In such a state your mind is in order and so is your relationship with your body and food.

Getting Flexible

To live in a non-personal way is to have a ball by being a ball. A ball can't be emotionally affected because, being round, it has no sides or positions to be partial to or prejudiced against. It's equal on all sides, the same all around. It can roll with equal ease in any direction the situation happens to be slanting. A ball can't land wrong-side up or upside down because it has no such distinctions or boundaries. When you're a ball, there's only one way you can ever land – right-side up. To be centered, then, is to be a ball; to be biased, is to be a square.

Being round enables you to roll with the punches of the world. Whenever you stand flatfooted or fixed, the slightest tap will rattle your brain or tip you over. In order to be unaffected by the world, your head and the world's fist must move, not toward each other, and not away from each other either, but in the same direction at the same time – more as if you were dancing rather than fighting. Life becomes a harmonious dance, not a conflicting struggle.

Given the hardness of the world and the softness of your head, wisdom demands a response to life that's a little more in tune with the world. To roll with the punches is not to compete with the world, but to cooperate with it, harmonize with it. When the orchestra is playing a tango, then dance the tango, not the Watusi; when at a funeral, be somber not cheerful. When at a wedding, be cheerful not somber. You don't tell the world what to do; the world, that is, the situation, tells you what to do.

My friend Maxie lost his job as waiter-trainee as a result of not understanding this principle of rolling or floating with the situation as opposed to being self-centeredly stuck in one position: He was balancing a large tray of fruit cocktails on one hand while serving them to guests with the other, when for the third time that evening the tray and dishes tipped over and crashed to the floor. When the manager came to investigate, Maxie explained that he was holding the tray at the exact center as he was told, but that after he had served two or three, the tray just tipped over by itself.

"But didn't you keep shifting your hand to compensate for the changing distribution of weight?" asked the manager. "Didn't you keep re-centering your position?"

"No," said Maxie, "I was trained to just hold the tray at its center."

"But the point of balance isn't a *fixed* point," said the manager, "It isn't a *particular* place. If the tray were empty, yes, the point of balance *would* be at its center, but the tray is not alone in the world; it lives in relationship with the dishes. So the center must be flexible to accommodate their spontaneous comings and goings. Every time a dish is removed from the tray it's a different situation, so you must move your hand to the new point of balance, the new center!"

"I didn't know you had to be an engineer to wait tables," replied Maxie.

That's when the manager politely asked Maxie to turn in his apron and leave the premises forthwith.

Self-centeredness operates under the misconception that *he* is the center of all experience, that everything revolves around *him.* In reality, the *situation* is the center, not you, personally. You are merely the actor, the player, the participant. The situation is the thing. Or in Shakespeare's words, "The play is the thing." You are nothing; the situation is everything. Again, the transaction is where the action is. Error is self-centered while detachment is situation-centered or neutrally-centered. Detachment has no self while the self-centered is full of himself, while detachment is free of himself and his appetite.

Now you don't want to eliminate, suppress or repress emotions because emotions are integral to health, clarity and happiness. What you do want to do is *control* them. Either you control them or they control you. There are no other choices. And the way you control them is to be relaxed *while* excited – another seeming paradox. Your usual pattern is to constantly bounce back and forth between excitement and relaxation like a ping-pong ball. Something moves you and *later* you calm down from it. Tension then calmness; then tension then calmness. Your goal now is to move the excitement part of the cycle and the relaxation part closer and closer together until they overlap or occur simultaneously. You want to be composed *as* you move, like a ballet dancer who can flit freely about the stage while maintaining a graceful and dignified poise every step of the way.

Being composed and excited at the same time is a process similar to that of walking up a down escalator where excitement is at the bottom, and relaxation is at the top. In order to stay centered between them, you have to move up at the same speed as the escalator is moving down. In this way you remain still *while* moving, calm *while* excited. In this way you can fully experience both the painful and the pleasurable without being negatively affected by either. When there's no discomfort, there's no reason or desire to overeat or eat for the wrong reason.

Getting Positive

The question becomes, what's your state of mind or feeling when you see all things with equal eyes? What's the prevailing mood when unaffected by neither pain nor pleasure? The feeling is one of *pleasure.* Whenever you're centered between opposing emotions, you automatically take on the *positive* one. When centered between doubt and confidence, you become confident; between resentment and acceptance, you become acceptant or forgiving; between guilt and innocence, you feel innocent, and likewise with all feelings. The positive always dominates with a balanced, centered attitude because it's the pole most compatible with your true nature, with reality. Human nature is essentially positive because conscious life in and of itself is a good and positive thing. Positive in that it's whole, compete, real, perfectly ordered, perfectly controlled. So to the degree you are centered in attitude, you become whole, complete, real, perfectly ordered and controlled yourself. You become compatible with life instead of at odds with it; consequently, the positive is what you'll naturally feel and express.

This principle is like the traffic law that says that when two vehicles approach an intersection at the same time (in balance), the one on the right (the positive one) has the right of way (becomes dominant). But when your perspective is imbalanced, you block out a part of yourself like a cloud blocks the sun. And in so doing, you become, in effect, un-whole, unreal, uncontrolled, disordered and stressed – and that's when you head for the refrigerator.

Now the sun isn't *really* gone; it's just blocked. This incompleteness or un-wholeness is felt as a negative deficiency or emptiness that you try to fill with food. Others try to fill it with sex, alcohol, gambling, shopping, etc. The thing to grasp here is that all such negativity is false. Negativity has no basis in reality. It's merely an appearance – an emotional optical illusion that's corrected when you *detach* from a personal, self-centered angle of vision to a more neutral or universal one. Think of negativity as a cup-shaped emotion. When you have this cup, you have to fill it with illicit food; when you don't have it, there's nothing that needs filling. So food's no longer a factor in your life.

A Double-Barreled Centering Technique

Staying relaxed and centered is a simple procedure of knowing what your present mood is, knowing what its opposite is, then moving between them by either *rejecting both* or *accepting both*. Let's say you're feeling angry toward someone. The opposite of anger is forgiveness, tolerance or acceptance. In *rejecting* both, don't accept the perceived offense and don't resent it either. Just remain the same, calm and composed – as if nothing happened. In *accepting* both, you resent and accept simultaneously, or as close together as possible. Here it's more obvious that nothing has changed, that you remain controlled and unaffected. So you don't have to eat over it. Or, in simpler terms, when you're angry, count to ten; when feeling depressed, start singing; when sad, start laughing; when bored, get curious; when doubtful, exude confidence, etc. Again, the subconscious mind is creative not logical. Contradict all negativity of any name or nature.

Overlooking the offense of others is, again, based on the reality that how a person behaves is *his* problem not yours. It's not any of your "personal" business. If a patient in an insane asylum insulted you, would you become upset? Of course not because you'd know the cause of his behavior is his mental imbalance and not you personally. Knowledge of his insanity would balance out the effect of the insult so you'd remain undisturbed. Now suppose an aggressive driver dangerously cuts you off on the highway, would you then react with anger? It would be inappropriate for the same reason as above – that the cause of the aggressiveness or rudeness is his problem not yours. It's a mental imbalance on his part and has nothing to do with you personally. The "sickness" here will of course be less obvious than in the above instance, but the difference is merely one of setting and degree – mental imbalance remains the case. You would respond appropriately but not with anger (or overeating). There's no emotional reaction to the *person,* but a composed response to the *situation.* The difference is that in the one case, you're out of control, and in the other, in control. In one case you're self-centered, in the other, *situation-centered.* In one case you took it personally, in the other, neutrally.

The rule of thumb is this: Whatever you say or do emotionally will tend to be the wrong response; whatever you say or do impersonally, will tend be correct and appropriate. Reacting with anger effectively makes you imbalanced too by pulling you away from your own center of poise. Through emotional reaction in general, and resentment in particular, the dis-ease of another is transferred to you. It becomes contagious. You complete the transaction some person, place or thing initiates. Something is being offered or suggested to you. You are being tested. You are being tempted. Will you accept? That's the question. It's attempting to sell you something. Will you buy? It takes two to complete a transaction. If you react emotionally, then you become its customer, its market. You put yourself in the same league with him or it. You are playing its game, on its level, and by its rules. He or it, consciously or unconsciously, is now controlling you, hypnotizing you, exploiting you, dominating you. You are not longer in possession of yourself; no longer your own person but have become subject to him or it. It acts and you re-act; it's the cause and you're the effected; it's the mover and you're the moved – straight to the refrigerator.

The world is like a glass windshield that has shattered into four billion interconnected people. The only difference among them is that each reflects "reality" at a slightly different angle. They're all of the same substance, but each expresses that substance according to his own unique, personal perspective. As far as higher consciousness is concerned, there are no good pieces or bad pieces, no right or wrong pieces. There are just *different* pieces. We come to realize that "reality" can't be seen with personal eyes, but only with impersonal, detached eyes.

Being a Mirror

The opposite of being a personality is being a medium or mirror. A mirror doesn't have any particular qualities or characteristics of its own. It simply reflects faithfully whatever is presented to it. The nature of a mirror is to be perfectly clear, for any blemish will affect the fidelity of its reflection. If it has any thoughts or beliefs of its own, then it'll no longer be an honest mirror but one that distorts everything it sees accordingly. If the mirror is to be effective, it cannot have a self of its own. It must be selfless; that is, it must have no opinions or concepts of its own in order to be able to see and reflect with total integrity.

Getting Creative

Thinking is an activity, and like desiring, it can be either emotional or creative. As a general rule of thumb, if thinking doesn't go somewhere in particular, doesn't contribute to solving a problem or achieving a conscious objective, then it's emotional. Hoping, trying, expecting, desiring, daydreaming, wishing, resenting, complaining, worrying, and the like, are emotional because they're of a negative, dead-end nature. They have no positive end. They just sit there sapping energy and giving nothing in return. Creative thought leads to and coincides with productive action. It brings problems and goals to resolution. There's no waste, no fat. Each thought pulls its own weight and contributes coherently to a moment to moment or overall plan. When you control thoughts and feelings, they become creative, and bring goals to fruition. When thoughts and feelings control you, creativity is stifled or blocked, and you experience frustration and failure.

The question to ask is, who's in charge here, you or your feelings? You are in control of your feelings because you can *observe* them. To be the observer is to be the controller, because the observer is *above* the things he observes; he's *superior* to them. You can objectively observe your thoughts, feelings and food issues, therefore, you can control them at will. You're not powerless over your food disorder to the degree you get above it, and you get above it by virtue of conscious detachment from all aspects of it.

The Law of Allowance

The law of allowance is related to the law of detachment. To allow or accept your disorder is to effectively separate or free yourself from it. You don't have to "do" anything in order to control your mind or eating. No mental activity is required. All that's necessary is the indifferent observation of it. To allow your disorder *is* to control it because then you're no longer emotionally entangled in it. You've let it go. You control it because you've removed the *conflict* that rendered you powerless over it. Conflict itself is the impotence factor; it's the killer of self-control power.

Letting Go

Letting go means dropping the idea that you can "think" yourself into control of your appetite or wrong eating behavior. Descartes said, "Perhaps everything we believe is false." If we're not living in detached reality, we're living in powerless ignorance, trance, or illusion. Our "thinking" gives us the false impression that we're in control. The more we "think" the more we imagine we are masters of our lives. The fact is, that apart from objective reality we are nothing; we have no *personal* control over our eating disorder whatsoever. The master of self-control said, "Of yourself (your lower self) you are nothing." – You can do nothing. To the degree you're tuned with objective reality, your disorder virtually corrects itself. Your "personal" knowledge, of itself, not only has nothing to do with it, but constitutes being out of order in the first place. It's what hinders recovery.

Everything you need to know to control your appetite and unwanted habits is within you right now and always has been. You don't have to reinvent the wheel. The universe has already been thought out for you. All you have to do is tap into it, flow along with it – and detachment is the way to do it. It's the means by which to let go of your lower self – which is the controllee not the controller.

Letting go is both difficult and easy – difficult in that, without all those positions and conditions about life and food that you've wrapped yourself in, you'd feel naked and vulnerable. But nakedness and vulnerability are the whole idea; they are the very essence of freedom. To be open and exposed means you have nothing to hide, nothing to defend, and therefore, nothing to fear or be anxious about, and nothing to eat over. All fear is the fear that, of yourself, you are nothing, compounded by the fear that others will discover it. The fact is that, of your (lower) self, you really are nothing and so is everyone else.

Letting go of personal defects is achieved by acknowledging them and accepting them. Then they drop by themselves. It'll be easy in the sense that you don't have to add anything to yourself, but rather, to drop things you've accumulated. We are all products of the same human condition. What you want to do now is to make the human condition a product of *you*. You do this by detaching from everything that's holding you against your will, whether from the past or in the present. To hold on to something takes energy and effort, but to release a thing requires neither – you just drop it. Separate from it. Disown it. Dis-identify with it.

Imagine that you're carrying all your knowledge (fat) in a shopping bag, years and years of accumulated information and misinformation are packed into it making it a very heavy load. To hold on to this bag day in and day out takes energy and effort, but to let it go, all you have to do is relax your hand. Release your grip and the bag (the fat) falls by itself.

If external information is so necessary to the control your life and your appetite, then how could you ever have enough of it? Where would it end? At what point would you consider your knowledge sufficient? If there is no end to it, there can't be a beginning either; that is, if you're deficient in something right now, then you'll always be. The book that would provide you with the knowledge needed to cope with this moment has not yet been written. And when it is, it will be immediately obsolete, for the situation that called for it will be gone, and the new situation will have a completely different set of variables, requiring yet another book that will also be obsolete on completion, and so on.

In other words, by depending on past knowledge to control yourself, you remain in the past yourself. You remain in a state of perpetual obsolescence. It's like being the trailer behind the car: The car is like reality, and the trailer is like the knowledge-dependent person who must always lag behind it.

The information necessary to handle this moment intelligently must come out of this moment, not out of the past – from within you, not from outside of you. Outside information is dead and gone; inside information (intuition) is alive and ever-present.

To be prepared to move in any direction with equal ease requires a mind that is open, empty, and still. A mind that contains anything at all will be restricted by those contents. Such a mind will not be able to "think on its feet" unless the questions that come up just happen to correspond with the predetermined answers it's carrying around. Which is unlikely, for reality does not conform to us; it is for us to conform to it. To have an answer without a question is just as useless as having a question without an answer.

Open-mindedness means not having any answers or any questions either; it's being totally empty so as not to impose limits on your own intelligence or common sense. Think of that bag of positions you're carrying as full of dead information like yesterday's newspaper. Pages and pages of dead answers to questions life is never going to ask again, and each answer having the effect of limiting or diminishing you a bit. Each premeditated answer uses up some of your intelligence like a computer's random access memory (RAM) is used up, so that at any given moment you're operating below speed and capacity. As you let the newspaper go when finished, so let the moment go when it's finished. Enter each new moment fresh, open, receptive. Keep your mind clear. Be ignorant like Socrates. Don't have any knowledge of your own, but be impartially interested in the knowledge of others.

The law of reverse effort applies to "believing" as well as to any other activity. You tend to be the opposite of what you think or believe. If you think you know it all, you know nothing; if you think you are wise, you are a fool; if you think you are educated, you are ignorant; if you think you are great, you are common; if you believe you're the life of the party, you are a bore, and so on. "Believing," in and of itself, indicates just the opposite – that you are doubting. Belief and doubt are two sides of the same mind, so that it's impossible to have a belief about something without also having a doubt about it.

To transcend this paradox, apply the "Double-Barreled Centering Technique." Depending on your personality, you can either believe everything or believe nothing; doubt everything or doubt nothing. Those are the only two choices that reality offers and no split orders, substitutions or exceptions are allowed. To let go, surrender, give up, all mean the same thing: to relinquish something lower so that something higher may operate. It means dropping the narrow, limited personality so that the higher potentiality within may work in its place. The intelligent organism that we are is what we're surrendering to. When through detachment, we give *in* or give *up,* it refers to our subconscious organism. When we go to sleep, we trust it, we give up to it; so why can't we do likewise when awake as well? Why can't we not give up to it when relating to our body and our food?

Being a Receptacle

In order to experience the reality of recovery from your eating disorder, you have to be receptive to it. Think of reality and yourself as two halves that join inside of you. Reality doesn't have a self or body of its own; it's "spiritual" like electricity and must live *through* you. Conversely, you don't have spirituality of your own but must live *from* it. We are merely receptacles into which this spirit may plug. Together we constitute reality; separate we exist as a powerless falsity. Just as a toaster isn't "really" a toaster until plugged into its source of power, so you aren't "really" a happy, intelligent and powerful human being unless plugged into your source of power – which is the subconscious mind.

When you're not "thinking," you're able to make direct contact with your body. Otherwise your stomach remains at arms length like a stranger – something with which you can never responsive and intimate. With a receptive and detached mind, you become fused to your body. You become consciously as well as organically connected to it like the head and tail of the same animal. It's only through being so connected with your body that you can know it and respond to it intuitively and immediately. Intuition is not emotional; it is essential common sense. It's operating with a clear conscience, a conscience unclouded and undisturbed by emotion.

Common sense is the ability to notice a pattern in what's going on and to spontaneously pinpoint the significance of it without having to *think* about it. When you see a work of art, for example, you know right off whether it "works," whether you like it. It correlates with your sense of harmony or doesn't. When listening to a piano recital and a wrong note is struck, you know it immediately, even without ever having heard the piece before or without any musical training. The same with your eating life: To the degree you're centered via detachment, you see your eating behavior with such acute clarity, that it becomes easy to stop or change it. It's only the incomplete picture of what you're doing to yourself and body that's been blocking your power to correct it.

Key Points and Principles to Remember from Chapter 6:

1. Being Centered is experiencing the ups and downs of life with total equanimity – allowing the world to swirl around outside of you, not inside of you;

2. Being Centered is like being the impartial juror at a trial, or the indifferent middle man in a business transaction;

3. Being Centered gives clarity and control of how you think, feel and eat;

4. Being Centered neutralizes the inner conflict about your eating behavior that renders you powerless over it:

5. Being Centered breaks the vicious circle where: stress blocks clarity, lack of clarity causes error, error results in failure, failure causes stress again;

6. Being Centered is being still while moving, relaxed while excited;

7. Allowing and accepting your body and behavior removes the conflict that renders you powerless over your body and behavior;

8. Being Centered relaxes the stress that triggers and feeds unwanted eating habits;

9. Being Centered via detachment, breaks the trance of your

eating habit;

10. Being Centered is the key to self-control, and detachment is the key to Being Centered.

CHAPTER 7

HOW TO CONTROL STRESS

"Control your emotions or they will control you." – Chinese proverb

Stress is public enemy number one. It's the root cause of most every preventable disease and unwanted condition that we experience in life. It negatively affects every part of our life – our health, happiness, clarity and appetite-control power. Managing stress is prerequisite to quality of life in general and to weight management in particular, so let it be the number one priority in your life.

Stress-control is based on the following logic: *If feelings of discomfort trigger your eating issue, then stop feeling discomfort.* Here we're treating both the cause and effect of the problem – knocking the whole ECH into oblivion along with any unhealthy or fattening behavior that came with it. Negative thoughts and feelings, such as of discontent, boredom, loneliness, anger, resentment, fear, doubt, guilt, uncertainty, worry, etc., control you more than logical thinking does. If you can't control these negatives, you won't be able to control much of anything else in your life – especially your appetite. Appetite-control *is* emotion-control and vice versa. Feel your feelings fully, both the negative and the positive ones, but don't let any take you over. Don't let any get under your skin. Oscar Wilde put it this way, "A man who is master of himself can end a sorrow as easily as he can invent a pleasure. I don't want to be at the mercy of my emotions. I want to use them, to enjoy them, and to dominate them."

The battle of the bulge is between impulse and restraint, desire and self-control, instant gratification and healthy delay. Resisting the impulse to eat when not hungry or to eat beyond satiety, is the root of emotional self-control. Think it through. Remember that when you choose a behavior, you choose the consequences.

Controlling Pain and Pleasure

We can greatly simplify the matter with the understanding that, in the whole world, there are only two emotions – negative ones and positive ones. For our purpose here, all other terms are academic. Names themselves don't matter; only their meaning matters. Emotion means movement; so "negative" means a backward movement – *away* from achieving your goal; "positive" means a forward movement – *toward* the achievement of your goal. But for communication purposes we'll name some of the emotions – the most important of which is *contentedness*, which we discussed in the Chapter 1.

True contentedness means that if your desires are not fulfilled, it doesn't make any difference to your happiness or well-being. If it doesn't make any emotional difference whether or not you lose weight, then you've already lost that weight or corrected the unwanted behavior; if it doesn't make any emotional difference whether or not you win, you've already won. This, again, is the

Law of Detachment, and is what being relaxed and centered is all about.

Contentedness means you are not deficient or lacking in anything. Nothing is missing from you. You are now complete and whole. You've reached to the understanding that, as Marcus Aurelius put it, "Everything is just as it is supposed to be." You have arrived. Whether you're a dishwasher or chairman of the board, it's only your contentedness that indicates that you are free and secure; that you have overcome the world.

Contentedness is indifference to both pleasure and pain. As far as your higher self is concerned, they are the same. You, the higher you, are unchanged, unfazed by either. You remain yourself – calm, composed, indifferent. Indifference means you are acceptant of what is. You don't (emotionally) desire that a situation be different than it is. You are pre-established in contentment. It is one of your most powerful pre-existing conditions. It's equal to bliss and love. Contentedness, then, is what transcends and controls pain and pleasure of any name or nature.

Pursuing Pleasure Produces Pain

The opposite of indifference is *emotional desire*. When you desire emotional pleasure through food, it means you've left the state of balanced relaxation and contentment, and negative feelings will be the inevitable result. There is nothing wrong, of course, with pleasure and gratification in and of themselves, it is the *desiring* part of the equation that causes the problems. Desiring is the emotional pressure that pulls you off balance and into the negative cause and effect, vicious cycle. Craving gratification is an emotional activity, and just like physical activity it's subject to the law of reverse effort that says "All action produces an equal and opposite reaction." So that whenever you seek gratification, you tend to get the opposite – pain, in the form of disappointment, frustration and failure. When you emotionally seek to lose weight, you tend to gain weight.

This principle also applies if you're experiencing pleasure right now and try to retain or cling to it. The clinging, like desiring, causes the pleasure to change to pain. But if you are experiencing pleasure and are indifferent to it – it remains. And the same is true of emotional pain. If you try to escape it, it persists, but if you experience it totally and indifferently, it changes to pleasure. Pleasure is relaxation, comfort and contentment. It indicates a state of joyous equanimity. Physical balance is the absence of physical pain, mental balance is the absence of negative thinking such as doubt or disbelief, and emotional balance is the end of emotional pain such as resentment, irritability or restlessness.

When you have no cravings or desires, you are relaxed and serene. Being relaxed and pain-free is perfectly natural. The proof that it's natural lies in the fact that when you are without pain you don't notice it, but if you have a worry, headache or desire, you're continuously uneasy. Pleasure is the norm. Pain is the aberration. When there's no pain, you just go happily about your business without thinking about it. You don't notice it. Peace and joy don't need a reason, but to suffer you need guilt, doubt, fear, etc.

Needing a reason to be happy is not natural; it indicates dis-ease. If you need a *reason* to be happy, then you can never be happy because the illusory deficiency that seeks for a reason now will remain with you always. As soon as you meet or are about to meet your criteria for "happiness" – immediately your seesaw of imbalance will pop up with yet another requirement, and then another. Your work is never rewarding enough. Life is never exciting enough. You never meet the "right" man or woman. You never have the money, possessions or security that you think you need to have. You never receive enough appreciation or recognition, etc. Applied to eating, you can never get enough food to sate the discomfort or fill the void. Discontent endlessly breeds further discontent. It's like trying to stabilize a rocking canoe, as soon as you move to one side, the other side wants to tip you. If you're looking for a *reason* to be happy, you'll always be looking. You'll remain a seeker and never a finder. Nothing will satisfy you. Everything will contain some insufficiency, some defect. Something will always be missing or falling just short of the mark. If you're not content with what is at this moment, then you can't be content with what should, would, or could be either. The only choice you have, then, is to be choiceless. It's to live in a state of total acceptance and allowance.

What is, is real; what should be is fantasy. Living in reality, in and of itself, is pleasing and gratifying. But living in accordance with how things should, would or could be, breeds endless frustration. If you're not happy in the rain, you can't be happy in the sun either for they are two sides of the same weather coin. In the first place, you cannot accept or reject only half a coin, and in the second place, the whole coin is irrelevant to happiness. Happiness is not dependent on one thing or another. It's totally self-sufficient. Like life, it doesn't come *from* things but exists in and of itself. Happiness is inherent not derivative. It's free-standing. Nothing external is needed. Happiness is just the way life is whether we like it or not, and has nothing to do with rain or shine, good or bad, right or wrong, fat or lean. So we have no choice but to like it. The attitude of reality is "Love it or leave it." When you overeat or under eat, you are leaving it.

Circumstances are just the props of life; just the scenery, setting or background. The backdrop is ever changing, but the real you, the authentic, relaxed you, remain always the same. One day you wear a blue suit, the next day a gray one; one day goes well, the next doesn't. Behind the suit and aside from the fluctuations in the market, you are the same person. The real, higher you cannot change, cannot become unhappy. Unhappiness is a dis-ease that doesn't occur in reality; it's something that's acquired, and we acquire it through emotionally desiring things be different from what they are right now. Life is neutral; it becomes a problem when we judge and criticize it; and it becomes joyous when lived indifferently and impersonally.

Pain Is an Imbalance Warning Signal

The purpose of physical, mental or emotional pain is to warn us that something unhealthy is going on. In health, the whole organism is working harmoniously; in disease, some imbalance or conflict is in effect, and pain is the means by which we're informed of it. If you're sitting on a hot stove, the pain would alert you to the danger. It's likewise with emotional pain such as that of anxiety or resentment. It's to remind us we're desiring something inappropriate or desiring in the wrong way.

So discomfort is really a positive thing; it's a friend not an enemy. It's not the problem itself but merely the messenger. Our mistake, of course, is that we try to kill the messenger instead of the *cause* of the problem. When there's physical pain we respond quickly and decisively. As soon as we notice the stove is hot we stop going there and are not likely to repeat the error. But emotional pain and tension are more subtle, not so compelling an emergency. So instead of seeking to understand and treat the cause, it's more expedient to just kill the messenger – which we attempt to do with various distractions, such as alcohol, drugs, sex, gambling, shopping, stock market, work, or food, etc.

Treating the symptom is quick and easy, but relief, if there is any, is superficial and fleeting. We want instant gratification but the side effects are often worse than the dis-ease itself. It's like instead of getting off the hot stove, you just sat there taking aspirins and tranquilizers – or trying a different diet program. The implication of all this is that maintaining a centered perspective or attitude is not a choice but a *law*. Yes, you do have the freedom of choice — to break or obey that law. But if you choose to break it, there will be a sure penalty — like an eating disorder. So you really don't have a choice. The universe is so structured that if you don't maintain an attitude of centered indifference toward people, places and things, you'll get burned.

Success is finding your own level, your own pace. It's to not go too fast, or be too ambitious, and it's to not go too slow, or be stagnant. It's to remain directly in the middle. Centered. The world turns at a certain speed and it's for you to find that speed. It's to "go with the flow." The pain of stress will be your foolproof guide. No need to rationalize or intellectualize it. Simply notice the exact moment when the tension or craving arises, then stop being affected by the feeling or stop doing what you're doing. Change the subject. And it's likewise while eating, notice when the hunger has abated then stop eating. When Pinocchio lied, his nose grew; when we lie or sin against our nature, our stomach grows.

Crying for The Moon

Tension comes from either desiring something you already have, as we discussed earlier, or desiring something you can't have. Let's say you see, in a shop window, a beautiful watch. You desire to own it *but* can't afford it right now. Just as the "but" splits the sentence in two, it also splits the mind in two. If you could afford that watch, you wouldn't *desire* it; you'd simply buy it! You'd see it, like it and buy it. There are no "buts" about it. No desire, conflict or stress is involved. The secret of contentment, then, is this: if you can have a thing, have it, but if you can't — don't desire it. In other words, don't desire what's not *already* yours. On the subconscious level you're already at your goal weight or behavior, so desiring it would backfire or short circuit your realizing that goal. It's like the first rule of closing a sale: When the prospect finally says yes to the salesperson's offer, the salesperson should immediately stop talking, because anything uttered thereafter would do nothing but jeopardize the sale. Mentally and emotionally you have already lost that weight, so stop desiring it. Only in this state of desirelessness can the weight-loss sale be consummated.

You can, however, *create* what is not yours. If you would have the watch you want or the body you want, then make it a creative activity instead of an emotional one. To desire is emotional – of a lower faculty; to create is spiritual. Longing for anything is incompatible with reality because, consciously or unconsciously, your organism already knows what all your needs and desires are and is already working toward their attainment. Whether or not you are aware of it, you are always heading in the direction of total fulfillment. The key is to just be more aware of your intention and more receptive to receiving it. All things being equal, your goal weight or eating behavior is already yours; it's already programmed into your genes. The whole task of detached intelligence is to just keep "all things equal," to just get out of the way and let nature run its course, to just follow the leading of common sense, and to not ignore it when tension reminds you that you've gone astray. You are, and have always been, the only hindrance to success. If you want to know what the problem, just look in the mirror. By desiring, you effectively contradict your own self, your own organism. It's like turning on the car's starter while the engine is already running, or driving with the emergency brake on. How frustrating and self-defeating. When tired, sleep; when hungry, eat. No desiring, dieting or willpower is involved.

The Law of Reversed Effort

According to Newton's Law, "All action produces an equal and opposite reaction." If you emotionally want to lose weight, you will gain more weight – as you've likely experienced. Emotional activity brings about the opposite of what we want by the same principle that propels a rocket or a jet airplane. In a balanced universe, movement one way *must* be compensated for by an equivalent movement the opposite way in order to maintain the balance. The plane's propulsion in one direction, propels the plane toward the opposite direction. So to make the plane go east, we aim the energy west. If we want the rocket to go up, we aim the energy down. And in the same way, if we want pain, we exert energy toward pleasure and gratification. But we can't apply this principle in reverse as the masochist attempts to do. We can't say, "I will then seek pleasure through pain." This doesn't work either, for seeking pain is just as ineffectual – long term, as seeking pleasure. Again, the problem is not *what* you emotionally seek but *that* you emotionally seek.

As you saw in Chapter 5, the universe turns in only one direction and that direction is neutral. If happiness and appetite control is your intention, then neutrality (being centered) is the direction you'd have to travel to get there. Think of a revolving door as the world. The door panel in front of you is "pleasure" – the pleasure of being your goal weight. The door behind you is "pain"– the pain of being overweight. When you push toward pleasure, pain (failure) comes right on your heels.

Now let's say the revolving doors are in motion. Perhaps there's someone in the compartment in front of you and someone in the one behind you. They're doing all the pushing. All you have to do now is to just go along for the ride. You don't have to push for pleasure but just remain neutrally centered by moving at the same speed the doors (the world) are moving.

This is a good example of creative movement where you are still and in action at the same time. You are moving but are still with respect to the doors. As far as the doors are concerned, you are not moving at all. The world is moving and you are moving with it. You are in unison. You and the world are not in conflict, not moving in different directions or different speeds but are equal in all respects.

A *Seesaw Named Desire*

Think of the world as a child's seesaw. One end is "pleasure," the other is "pain," and you – the higher you, are situated at the center. The seesaw is in perfect balance; that is, until you begin to step out in the direction of "pleasure" causing it to fall and "pain" to simultaneously rise up to become dominant.

Desiring is like trying to remove a speck from your soup. As you approach the speck with your spoon, it slips away, and the faster you chase it, the faster it moves away. The only way to catch it is to chase it creatively rather than emotionally. Instead of *moving* after it, be *still* and let it come to you. Be receptive – by lowering the spoon to just below the surface (the subconscious) of the soup, so the speck flows into the spoon naturally, by gravity. Thus, you attain it without chasing it. The speck wasn't the problem; the approach was the problem.

The reason the speck eludes the spoon so naturally is because they are physically connected so have no choice. The soup is the medium connecting spoon and speck. It's the physical link that also separates them. Just as a car and its trailer stay separate by virtue of the hitch between them, so the spoon and the speck stay separate by virtue of the soup between them.

The way it works physically is the way it works emotionally: Pain and pleasure are directly linked but we don't notice the connection because it's so subtle in the same way that we don't notice the soup as a connective because it's so un-solid or unsubstantial. Thus pain and pleasure are connected as two sides of one continuous mind. They're a continuum. If you emote toward pleasure you come to pain; if you try to escape, it follows like a shadow.

Your only alternative is to transcend the whole coin. Rise above it by living on the center of the coin instead of on either surface of it. By remaining at the center, the point and attitude of detached indifference, you experience natural pleasure *all* of the time instead of emotional (false) pleasure *some* of the time. Your appetite comes and remains under effortless control. Pounds drop in due course.

Attachment to Pleasure Changes it to Pain

If you're experiencing pleasure while eating and try to prolong that pleasure by eating beyond satiety – you quickly lose it. Just as emotional effort toward pleasure causes pain, so does trying to hang onto the pleasure you're experiencing also causes pain. Clinging to anything is, in effect, an attempt to deny what is. A person finding a slice of chocolate cake delicious and gratifying would like to hang onto that pleasure, so she has another slice. But the second slice is not quite as good as the first, and the third is about to make her ill. What was delicious a few slices ago has become a virtual poison. Clinging attachment caused what was sweet to turn sour, not because the *cake* had changed each time, but because the *situation* had changed each time. Attachment rather than detachment caused what was beautiful to quickly become ugly.

Indifference to Pleasure Causes it to Remain

If you can experience the *sensual* pleasure of food without being emotionally affected by it, then there will simply be no need or desire to overeat. When you don't get excited about anything, especially food, you are then simply being yourself – happy and content. When you're content, your mind is still like a placid lake; when excited, it ripples in agitation. It was relaxed and centered, but your emotional response disturbed it, affected it. So by remaining unmoved or unchanged by the beauty, smell and taste of the food, the sensual pleasure doesn't change either. You eat when the body is hungry and stop when the hunger subsides. Happiness and appetite-control are enjoying food without attachment – without getting anything out of it but physical nourishment and sensual pleasure. And that is quite enough.

Escaping Pain Causes it to Persist

Running from discomfort doesn't work for the same reason chasing gratification doesn't work – they're both emotional activities and anything emotional must, by law, backfire. They are, in effect, equally negative. In desire we get the opposite of what we want; in escape we get more of what we're trying to escape from. This principle can be seen in the same revolving door illustration used earlier. There we saw that in pushing the pleasure of food, we caused pain to come upon us. Here, by pushing the front door forward in order to escape the pain-door behind us, we find the pain-door follows us like a shadow. The actions in both cases are the same, only the motives are different. And both are doomed to failure, again, not because their motives are right or wrong but because both are emotional rather than creative.

Whatever we try to escape, avoid, resist or suppress – we endow with power. Emotional discomfort, in and of itself, has no power to harm us; it is merely a signaling device, an indicator, a messenger. By avoiding the messenger we, in effect, make the messenger the issue instead of the imbalance it represents. The messenger then mistakenly becomes the evil with which we have to deal. It becomes what we must escape, resist, struggle with or kill. It's what we must drown with alcohol, kill with drugs, engorge with food, distract with excitement, etc. But this error is insidious and insatiable. A bottomless pit.

When you attempt to treat the symptom rather than the cause, nothing works. The ego is stubborn and foolish. It refuses to see and admit its error, refuses to see that it's self-centered perspective is a false one. So it spends its life in denial, trying to avoid the truth or trying to prove a lie is the truth. Here you can see the need for rigorous self-honesty if you are to win this battle.

In this we see the basic difference between the creative and the emotional: The creative lives in truth; the emotional lives in a lie or in fantasy. The creative is at peace; the emotional is disturbed. The creative comes from contentment; the emotional comes from hunger.

Accepting Pain Changes it to Pleasure

When you allow and accept the pain you're experiencing, that pain naturally converts to pleasure. The most effective remedy for handling emotional discomfort is simply to experience it fully and indifferently. To the degree discomfort is allowed rather than rejected, it disappears. The positive attitude of acceptance cancels or neutralizes the negative discomfort. It balances it out of existence. It transcends it, corrects it.

Emotional agitation is relaxed simply by virtue of the still, passive, detached awareness of the agitation. The agitation relaxes by itself. When we're experiencing discomfort without "desiring" that it should leave or without attempting to escape it (escapism), we're then in a state of centered indifference in which discomfort cannot exist. And if discomfort doesn't exist, neither does the need to overeat.

Emotional discomfort becomes obsolete simply through the indifferent allowance and acceptance of it. In other words, to eliminate anything negative or unpleasant we move *into* it not away from it. We confront it rather than resist it. Pain and pleasure are a single continuum like the inside of the cup that continues to the outside of the cup. By entering the pain we eventually come to the pleasure, just as by entering far enough into the night the day must appear. As night becomes day, so does pain become pleasure. If feeling depressed, for instance, you'd do nothing about it except witness it indifferently. You wouldn't like it, hate it, want it to stay or want it to leave, but would indifferently observe it out of existence.

The word *pain* comes from the Greek and Latin meaning *penalty*. Pain is the penalty we pay for violating the Law of Detachment. Whenever there's discomfort, whether from boredom, guilt, worry, resentment, anxiousness, depression, doubt, fear, uncertainty, etc., just allow it. Think of it as just a temporary aberration. Don't interfere with it in any way. The negativity came from emotional involvement in the first place. To reverse the process, we don't want to feed it more of the same. To reverse the process, our relationship with negativity of any name or nature, has to be one of detachment from it, not one of entanglement or engrossment in it.

Appreciating Your Pain

You allow and accept your discomfort knowing that its sole purpose is to lead you back to the truth that would free you from it. To appreciate a thing is to totally experience it. Any discomfort experienced to the end must leave you. There's simply no place for pain to gain a foothold. Whenever tension arises, don't be averse to it but enter into it. Relish it as an opportunity to regain more or your lost joy, freedom and control. Look it straight in the eye with calm, firm, detached indifference and watch it vaporize out of existence. Passive, creative energy works like a light that makes the dark disappear. As darkness is merely the absence of light, so pain is merely the absence of objective awareness. By shining impartial attention on pain or craving, you expose its nothingness, its superficiality. The two can't exist simultaneously.

Contentment is the total acceptance of people, places and things just as they are. We have to relate to everything if we are to relate to anything. And likewise, we have to accept ourselves in our totality as well. We're just as complex as the world is, the product of countless generations – and perhaps lives, of evolutionary development. Everything we ever were is within us now, and everything we'll ever become is also within us now. We consist of so many conflicting thoughts, feelings, attitudes and beliefs, that the only way to relate to them all is to indifferently accept them all. Otherwise, we'd become insane or neurotic – like a centipede trying to figure out which leg to use next.

You don't have to understand all things at all times. If you are feeling jealousy, sadness, resentment, hate, greed, loneliness, boredom, cravings, etc., allow it. Accept it. At those moments, that's what you are. To deny with guilt, regret or shame is disordered thinking that will lead to other disordered eating. Remember the Serenity Prayer: "God, grant me the serenity to accept the things I cannot change, the courage to change the things I can, and the wisdom to know the difference."

Any discomfort you repress or suppress becomes a toxin that will taint your whole being. It will negatively color all that you say, think, feel and do. Emotional eating means something is eating you. Think of negativity as a mental or emotional bacteria that eats you to the degree you are attached to it. Attachment gives it a septic home or foundation from which to fester into fat or disease. When you are detachedly aware of your anger, the anger is controlled – period. It's like the effect of "counting to ten." It subsides. It *must* subside. Detachment is the controlling factor. Anger is a neutral energy, but becomes explosive when repressed. When anger or resentment is thus controlled, your appetite becomes controlled – nullifying the desire to eat beyond satiety.

Remember the distinction that negative feelings are *what* you are, not *who* you are. Who you are is the pure, detached awareness that's above it all.

Creating Your Own Monsters

If you emotionally desire, try, wish, hope to succeed at controlling your appetite, then you will fail. It cannot be otherwise for again, they are two sides of the same mind. If you would be happy and successful, then be so. Why bring desire or effort into the picture? By desiring you introduce a conflict into the equation that doesn't exist. You, in effect, make struggle a foregone conclusion before even beginning. You create resistance by anticipating it. To fight something is to feed it. That's the meaning of the saying, "Resist not evil." You create an adversary relationship between you and your goal that's fictitious. Your goal doesn't care if it's attained by you or not. It's totally indifferent to your designs on it. It's just sitting there to be or not be partaken of. By desiring, you place it on a pedestal and give it artificial prominence. The more emotional the desire the greater the prominence. You set yourself up to fail by creating blocks where none exist. For every desire there *must* also be a complementary block built into it. Where there's no block there's no desire, and where no desire, no block.

In reality you can' desire and you can't try; you either have it or don't. The only question to ask yourself, then, is whether you have it. If not, no amount of desire and effort will help. A flower doesn't desire or use effort to grow; it simply grows. It has a direction but not a desire. A desire is emotional and failure prone, while direction is creative and success prone. The flower's "goal" is pre-determined and inherent, so doesn't need to desire. It's virtually already where it's going. It's just a matter of time. The purpose of a flower is to bloom to its full potential. And its source of power is the sun. Now all it has to do is let go and be itself in the direction of its source — and creation happens of its own accord. "Spring comes and the grass grows by itself," is the Zen saying. No emotional desire, effort or ego ambition is involved. It's just being itself, and to just be is to spontaneously flower. It just relaxes, and out of that stillness, out of that holy indifference it joyously blooms into the richest colors and the sweetest perfumes. So the pounds drop by themselves.

Living in reality is understanding that, to some degree or other, we're indeed personally biased with respect to practically all that we think, feel and do, and as a result, lose some degree of clarity and power. Descartes put it this way: "Perhaps everything we believe is false." It's not a question of maybe we are biased or to what degree, but that we are. Being present in the flesh, in and of itself, implies the existence of a self-centered bias. The point is that we don't *have* a bias, we *are* a bias. The eyes can't see themselves because the eyes are the things doing the seeing. The nose can't smell itself for the same reason, and so on with all the senses. And likewise with thoughts and feelings. Thoughts can't think of themselves and feelings can't feel themselves. That's the blind spot of clarity and power. That's the existential handicap we have to overcome. We overcome it by getting outside of ourselves, getting above ourselves. *We have to be on the outside looking in as well as on the inside looking out*. That's what detachment is, and that's how you get above an eating disorder and all the stress and negative feelings that trigger and trail it.

Think of yourself as a business organization with your thoughts, feelings and five senses serving as your seven key employees, and you are the objective overseer. The thinking faculty does all the planning and organizing for you. It's the brains of the organization, the computer. The body is your eyes and ears, and also does all the legwork for you. The feelings inform you whether things are going as planned. And you, the higher awareness, remain above them all, and by virtue of your aboveness, you control them all.

The way the employer maintains control is by keeping an appropriate distance from his employees so that their respective roles don't conflict. You allow them to play their roles without influencing or affecting their report; and likewise, you don't allow their report to personally (emotionally) influence or affect you. In this way, the parts work together for the good of the whole. They are independent and in harmony at the same time. Everything's under natural and effortless control. When your mind is so organized and ordered, so will be your appetite.

Increasing Detachment

Controlling the mind is nothing more than being detachedly aware of its activity. By observing thoughts from a distance you control those thoughts. Nothing else has to be done. Detached awareness, in and of itself, is the controlling factor. You are not desiring to stop, repress or change the mind by force, but just to witness it as it is. By simply witnessing it, you control or change it.

Mind/body activity is like a child at play. To control him, we don't have to bridle him; we just watch him. Watch is controlling. He can't begin to get into mischief because we're right there, right on top of the situation – above it all. The same with the mind: negative or misleading thoughts or feelings can't begin to harm you because you're above them at the moment of their inception. By observing mind/body activities in a detached way, it becomes obvious that they, in and of themselves, have absolutely no power over you. You needn't be controlled by either negative or positive feelings. As far as your higher awareness is concerned, they are *just* feelings. That's what being relaxed, centered and free is, and that's what your true nature is.

Know Thyself

Socrates condensed all wisdom into two words: "Know thyself." If you know how your mind/body works, it's much easier to control yourself. If you don't know how you tick, you just repeat the same error indefinitely. To know yourself is to detachedly observe your lower self, your lower faculties. By witnessing thoughts, feelings and behavior from a distance, you see *first hand* who you are and why you eat as you do.

To the degree possible, notice all mental activity. Just pay attention to it as it is whenever it occurs. Know that you're thinking whenever you're thinking. When thinking about going to a restaurant, *know* that's what you're thinking. When playing tennis and thinking you might win or lose, witness yourself thinking those thoughts. When reflecting on a problem at work, watch yourself thinking the matter over and deciding on a course of action. When you find yourself daydreaming or musing, catch yourself doing it. Are you thinking of what you'll wear, what you'll say, what might be the response to what you say? Thinking of hurting someone, helping someone? Thinking about money, food, sex, reading, writing, retirement? Be aware that you are. And even when there's no thought activity at all, be conscious of that too. By persistently and choicelessly witnessing your thoughts and feelings in this way. you'll soon break the false identity or attachment you have with those thoughts and so regain control in the process. It will become clear that you're indeed above and in control of your thoughts. Once you know you can control your thoughts, you'll know that you can control your whole life. This is not about being self-conscious, it's about being *higher* self-conscious.

Your attitude with respect to all feeling is that they're all alike; they're all the same to you. One feeling is just as good or bad or right or wrong as any other. You don't feel guilty about the one, nor saintly about the other. From the perspective of a detached, impartial observer, there's no difference between a negative feeling and a positive feeling; they'e both just feelings. In other words, "No matter how you slice it, it's still baloney." The rule of thumb is this: if it's a mental activity, no matter how lowly or noble, it's not real but a concept or an illusion. It may or not become real later, but at this stage, it's just imagination. And it's just this detachment that'll give you the power to wisely discriminate between which thoughts you'll discard, and which you'll convert to actuality.

Increasing Emotional Awareness

You control feelings the same way you control thought, by observing them from a distance. By witnessing your feelings without letting them get under your skin, you effectively correct the wrong relationship you've been having with them. You put emotion back in its proper place – as the employee not the employer, as the subordinate not the superior. Feelings are to inform not to control. When a feeling arises for or against something, whether negative, positive, painful or pleasurable, do not react to it in any way, but just witness it with calm disinterest and humility.

If some person, place or thing is irritating you, just observe the fact of that irritation and nothing else. You're not concerned with whether the irritation is justified – you're not a judge; you're only concerned with the fact that it *exists.* If irritation is what you're feeling in that moment, just acknowledge, admit and accept it. Also acknowledge that it's not *you* that's irritated; it's the *feelings* that are irritated. The "you" are above them. Then, by virtue of the laws of allowance and detachment, the negative ones will leave, and the positive ones will remain.

If you can stand back and witness the irritation from a distance, you'll see that the irritation originated with you – the lower you. It was of your doing, your responsibility. You did it to yourself by owning or identifying with the feeling. You made the feeling who and what you are. Your feelings have taken you over, and an outside agency is pulling the strings or pressing the buttons. Instead of observing the situation from a distance, you became personally, emotionally, egotistically involved. You violated the integrity of whatever role you happened to be playing at the time. You took a social, business or family situation and personalized it. If a person acts improperly, it's not your personal concern; it's the concern of your *role* to respond accordingly. If you were a judge and were provoked by a lawyer, you'd hold him in "contempt." The contempt the judge "feels" is not personal but official. In the same way, if your child's behavior is "out of order," the matter would be handled parentally not personally. Likewise in any relationship. The offended party would not react personally, but in a manner appropriate to the role and situation. More on this in the Chapter 8, *How to Act.*

Reality is not concerned with whether you're feeling sad or happy, bored or excited, guilty or innocent, doubtful or confident, angry or forgiving. As far as reality is concerned, they're all the same; they're just feelings. Reality is like a cup – totally indifferent to what's poured into it. It doesn't accept one beverage over another, but is equally receptive to and unaffected by whatever is poured into it. Similarly, a flashlight doesn't shine more on some things than others; it shines equally on everything. And a flashlight doesn't change according to what it shines on either. Both the beautiful and the ugly have no affect on it. It remains true to itself – just an impartial, detached flashlight. If we can remain in reality by adopting the attitude of the cup or the flashlight, all fear and conflict would be eliminated, and along with it, the false need to overeat – or to starve.

Fear is always of the unknown, and conflict is always of one feeling or thought against its opposite. If you understand that life consists of nothing but negative and positive thoughts and feelings, then you know all there is to know. And if you know that the negative and positive are exactly alike, as far as your higher consciousness is concerned, then there can be no conflict. You know all there is to know, and you know how to respond to it. There's nothing else. You've got it. Now you're free. Now you're really educated and cultivated – no longer ignorant. You know universal convention and can move within it with freedom, ease and confidence. Now you can relax and enjoy life and food without getting carried away by either.

Whatever comes into your cup, whether pleasant or unpleasant, embrace it without judgment. Don't wrestle with it, argue with it, or entertain it in any way. Do not love it, hate it or fear it. Don't accept or reject it; but just be indifferently aware of it. You're playing the role of a cup and the appropriate behavior for a cup is to not get attached to the contents, but to keep a conscious distance from them. Don't allow your contents to push or pull you or raise or lower you; but remain firmly in the center of them. Neither indulge nor repress them – just witness them from a distance. (When you're witnessing you're discriminating; when attached, you are judging. One is of the higher self, the other, of the lower self.) When you thus break the identification with your contents (your lower faculties), you're no longer subject to them. They become subject to you. *You're no longer subject to the world; the world (your body) becomes subject to you.* You no longer react robotically to anything past or present. Your eating-for-comfort program is nullified.

Key Points and Principles to Remember from Chapter 7:

1. That stress is the trigger and fuel for virtually every unwanted eating behavior;

2. That you can control stress by keeping a conscious distance from all negative thoughts, feelings and activities;

3. That the emotional pursuit of pleasure produces pain;

4. That attachment to emotional pleasure causes pain;

5. That indifference to emotional pleasure causes it to

remain; That trying to escape from emotional pain causes it to remain.

CHAPTER 8

HOW TO ACT

"All the world is a stage and all the men and women, merely players." – Shakespeare

The "How to Act" Principle

Shakespeare's statement is not just clever metaphor; it is literal truth. The Law of Detachment applies not only to being above all that you think, feel and eat; it also applies to being above all the roles you play – for the same reason: Being above and distinct from the roles you play is the way to control yourself and your behavior. It's living in reality. Just as your thoughts, feelings and senses are not *really* you, so the roles you play are not *really* you. They're just acts you perform on occasion. The real you are consciously above them all.

Here again, to know yourself is to control yourself and your appetite. This "truth" of what you really are is the controlling factor. Understanding the distinction between who you are and how to act resolves the conflict that diminishes power over your life.

When you know yourself in this sense, you know virtually everything. Nothing else needs to be done but to practice keeping a respectable distance from the personal roles you play – including the role of yourself as a consciously detached eater. When you see eating as just another "role" to be played, you tend to play it more mindfully and meaningfully. It becomes a meditation. You're on the outside looking in at your eating instead of being mindlessly mired in it.

The "Situation is Everything" Principle

How does one "act" in an emotionally-controlled, conflict-free way? The answer is by *letting the situation determine your role, and letting the role determine your behavior.* The "situation" is the relationship in which you find yourself at any given moment, and your "role" is the particular part you play in that relationship, such as employer/employee, clerk/customer, husband/wife, parent/child, professional/client, etc., and correct behavior is that which is *appropriate* to that role.

Thus you act, but not according to your personal bias or ego; you act according to a role determined by the *situation. Your ego has been effectively detached from the decision-making process.* There's no longer a conflict of personality. You now act according to the fact of the situation rather than the biased opinion of the personality. You act according to principle rather than caprice.

To the degree you do, you live confidently instead of insecurely. Calmly instead of tensely. You become more free-flowing, more actual, more yourself. You move from role-to-role with the ease and grace of a ballerina rather than the fearful studiedness of an automaton. And the beauty of it is, you don't have to think about it; it's all unpremeditated, all unstressful. Freedom means decisions are simpler, less complicated. You become more decisive. And all you have to do is know the situation you're in, know your role in it, then *act* accordingly to the best of your ability.

Keeping Your Distance

All parties in a relationship have a certain role that determines how each is expected to behave. In order for society to function in an orderly and efficient way, it's members must act in conformance with certain conventions of behavior. The clerk is expected to behave in a certain way with respect to his customer, and the customer, with respect to the clerk. And likewise in the relationships between professional and client, teacher and student, parent and offspring, husband and wife, employer and employee, etc. Each has an obligation and responsibility to act towards the other in a manner characteristic of the role being played.

Being in Relationship

As our subject is "acting," it'll be useful to think in theatrical or literary terms. Think of yourself as the main character in a play. You, the protagonist, are the person around whom the play or story revolves. You're the center of the action, the center of attraction. But you're not there alone, not there in a vacuum; you're there and you act in relationship with the person, place or thing in the scene with you. You are never really alone, never really not in relationship with someone or something. In one scene you're at home with your family and playing the role of "husband" or "wife" with respect to your spouse, or "mother" or "father" with respect to your children. In another scene, you're at work playing the part of a "co-worker" with respect to other co-workers, or the alternating roles of "manager" to your subordinates and "subordinate" to your managers. In other scenes, you are playing the role of a "spectator" at a performance, "participant" at a social gathering, "friend" with respect to a friend, and so on. Even when alone you're playing a role such as a "listener" with respect to music, a "viewer" with respect to television, a "reader" with respect to your newspaper, a "diner" with respect to eating, etc. These scenes are the ever-changing backgrounds, settings and contexts in which you, the central character, perform.

In all these scenes, you're there in relation or connection to someone or something else. Even when alone, you are relating to yourself, to your higher self's consciousness or to your lower self's thoughts, feelings and desires. In a universe where all things are connected, it's impossible *not* to be related to something at any given moment. The key to good acting is always knowing what is that person, place or thing. If you don't know how your presence is immediately pertinent to a situation, you can't know what your proper role is or how to play it correctly. You won't know how to act. You'll feel insecure about your acting ability. Clarity and power over yourself, therefore, come from thinking of all situations in terms of *relationships.* So when you're eating, you're in a relationship with food – with you the controller, and food the controlee.

The Role is Real

Once reality is understood as a relationship, it becomes obvious that the role you play in it is also "real" – not *absolutely* real, but real in the sense that it's compatible and consistent with how to function in the world, how to function in harmony with the world so as to be in "control" of it. Roles are not you in the higher spiritual sense; they're you in the lower, personal sense. In the spiritual sense your "identity" never changes; you are always the impersonal observer *above* everything including all the roles you play. On the personal level, your identity must constantly change to accord with the situation or circumstance. Thus, by "playing a role" you *are* being real; you are being in tune with reality. To not play a role is to live in error and powerlessness.

Put another way, your role is not *who* you are; it's what you do. It's your work, duty, function, position, or office. A "judge" is not *really* a judge but just *acts* a judge when "on the bench." When he leaves the courthouse, he no longer acts as judge but as "husband" to his wife, "father" to his children, etc. And likewise, "parents" are not *really* parents in the higher sense, but just play the role of parents. That a role comes by way of a biological relationship rather than a social or business one does not make it any less a role to be detachedly played.

Reality does not differentiate between biology and society. All roles, regardless of their level or genesis, must be played in the orderly and principled manner appropriate to them. To the degree they are, there is harmony and control; to the degree they are not, there's conflict. The conflict comes from the false identity of confusing who you are with what you do. You are both a human being and a human doing. Being is who you really are;

doing is just an act, just a transient part you play.

The difference is one of perspective. Before, you didn't think in terms of "playing a role" because you were so self-centeredly identified with everything you did, that you believed you actually *were* all the parts you played. You couldn't separate the actor from the act – which is a form of insanity, like the person convinced that he's Napoleon. So the difference between conscious and unconscious role-playing is that in the one case, you emotionally identify with your role – you think it's really you; and in the other case, you see yourself as separate from it, above it, detached from it. You see your role merely as a human convention, just a "hat" to be worn; not as something to take personally, but as something to be taken creatively or recreationally.

The role itself is artificial but your act is real. You are the artist, and your role is your medium. Playing a role doesn't mean you are not yourself; on the contrary, you are fully yourself, but *you are yourself in the context of your role.* The role provides the necessary vehicle or means by which you *can* express yourself authentically. To be authentic simply means to be uniquely yourself. And since you already are yourself – and cannot be anything other no matter how much you try, all that remains is to have some vehicle or platform from which to express. Your family, social, business and professional roles provide that platform. If you are playing the role of a waiter, business person, housekeeper, artist, doctor, clerk, parent – it's your own unique personality that distinguishes you from all others playing the same role. Your role, like the body in which you live, is superficial, but the personality that animates and gives it expression, is authentic – and that's the source of your personal power.

The Real Actor Can Play Any Role

The mark of an authentic actor is his adaptability. He can move with equal ease into any role, while the bad or false actor is limited in the types of roles he can play. The false actor is like a painter who can paint landscapes but not seascapes, or like a novelist who can write mysteries but not romances, or like a salesperson who can sell oranges but not apples. These are not real artists. A real painter can paint anything, a real writer can write anything, a real salesperson can sell anything. In whatever situation you find yourself, what matters is that you're real, and being consciously an actor is *how* to be real, is the *method* of being real. Where there's no personality disorder there's no eating disorder.

The authentic actor has the flexibility of a chameleon. A chameleon's color is not fixed, but changes in accordance with his environment. When on a brown tree, he turns brown; when on a green leaf he becomes green. If you asked him what color he is, he could only say, "It depends on the situation." Or, if he was a sales chameleon, he might say, "What color do you want?" Similarly, when the authentic actor is in Rome, he dances the Tarantella; when in Tel Aviv, he sings *Havah Nagilah*. If he's poor, he does without; if rich, he lives lavishly. When at a wedding banquet, he plays the "celebrant"; at a funeral, he becomes a "mourner." *Knowing how to act is knowing how to live.*

If the chameleon didn't change colors he'd stand out, exposing himself to danger. Likewise, if a person was cheerful at a funeral and somber at a wedding, he too would stand out and be in danger – of being shunned by his fellows. He would not be in harmony with the situation, not be "one" with it. We say such a person doesn't know how to act, doesn't know his part. He's an outcast, isolated from the situation rather than related to it. This isolation makes him a stranger instead of a participant. He may not like the situation he's in, but that's beside the point. As an actor, that's none of his business. The point of fact is, he's there, so is obliged to act accordingly. Likes and dislikes are emotional considerations – not part of the real actor's persona. They are irrelevant to the reality of the situation and one's role in it. The real actor is only concerned with what is, and that his response is *equal* to it.

The Service Principle

The authentic actor doesn't have a "self" from which to like or dislike. He has no passions, feelings or desires of his own ego. He's just an actor, just a selfless medium. Whatever he feels is not for himself, but for his role. He feels with the situation or person he's with. If you're hurt, he's hurt; if you're happy, he's happy. Whatever you want is what he wants; wherever you want to go is where he wants to go. His being is virtually determined by you. You're the director of the play. For of himself he is already fulfilled, already "there," so has no need to do anything else but to give or serve.

So this "serving" is more than just a "good" thing, it's a *law* based on the fact that when you're above it all, there's nothing left to do but give. A servant is what you are and what you do. It's your *modus operandi*, your underlying motive in all relationship.

Conscious and constant service to others is the love/wisdom-based method of transforming from self-centeredness to other-centeredness. Service is the natural method or "technique" for getting out of yourself, for expressing your self. You are a "method" actor, and service is your secret, all powerful method of expression.

This explains why we feel good when we donate to charity or help a person or animal in need. Even the simplest thing like giving directions to a lost driver makes us feel good. Why? Because *serving is the fulfillment of our purpose in life*. It's the essential expression of the selfless soul.

Service is regarding and appreciating others. A basic human need is to be appreciated for who we are. We're all special in that there's no one in the world quite like us. While being different is nothing of which to be "proud"; it is something to be recognized. People *are* different. Relating to them, therefore, implies relating to their differences. If we are to connect to a person at all, we must recognize, understand and appreciate that person. There's no other way. To be with someone and not appreciate his uniqueness is to not *really* be with him except on the most superficial and meaningless level. Appreciating and recognizing the specialness of others is correct and good, and we certainly *will* benefit from it – for giving is the way of getting, but that's not why we do it. We do it because it's essential to authentic relationship and the fulfillment of being.

We respect a person by being sensitively aware of his presence. Awareness and sensitivity require energy, and merely applying energy to a person, in and of itself, is being respectful and appreciative. It's to listen with undivided attention – not listening with your mind elsewhere, or listening and casting judgment, or listening with an ear to how this person may be useful to you. You are listening for the purpose of understanding that person, understanding how *you* can be of use to that person – nothing else. The authentic actor lives in a service-based relationship with others, while the false actor lives in a self-based, self-centered one – then overeats to relieve the resulting boredom and loneliness.

This Principle of Service applies professionally as well. To the degree you think of benefitting the client first rather than yourself first, you'll be far more effective in "selling" both your product, service or idea.

Relationship Integrity

All roles are "professional" in that they are played, not according to personal feelings, but to the dictates of the role itself. And as there's never a time when you're not playing some role)except when sleeping(, there's never a time when you act according to uncontrolled feelings. Keeping a respectable distance between one another's role means we respect the sanctity of both the individual and the role he's playing. We respect the inviolable privacy of the individual. We don't get too familiar with anyone and don't allow anyone to get too familiar with us. "Familiarity breeds contempt" because it violates privacy and the integrity of the relationship. To have our privacy or "space" invaded is to have our soul or center taken over so that we're no longer our secure selves but are now being used or exploited.

Friendship is only appropriate between friends, not between buyer and seller, employer and employee, parent and child, etc.

We respect each other's role and privacy. The same applies within the family; we regard each other's privacy through behaving in strict conformance to role. The father and mother guide and nurture; the children listen and obey. The family, as in any successful organization or government, works according to a hierarchy of one leader, one second, one third, etc. Any reversal of roles, such as the children controlling the parents or the mother acting as the head instead of the father, will cause a breakdown in the family, as it would in any organization. The sergeant obeys the captain, the worker is subservient to the manager, and so on; otherwise the relationship doesn't work. It becomes dysfunctional.

Of course, the head of the household, for example, must act in a manner appropriate to that position. He can't use that "official" position for his own personal gratification, but only for the good of the family as a whole. With position comes responsibility. The French term *noblesse oblige* means the "head" has an obligation and responsibility to act in a way that befits such a role. It's for your wife and children to respect your role, but it's for you to be unfailingly worthy of that respect by playing it appropriately.

The same principle applies to food. We keep a respectable and emotional distance from food so as not to violate the integrity of the relationship – and overeat as a consequence. The role of the eater is, again, to eat for physical purposes not emotional purposes.

Key Points and Principles to Remember from Chapter 8

1. That in order to control yourself, you have to know yourself;

2. That to know yourself is to know your role in every situation;

3. That there's no time when you're not playing a role;

4. That you are above and distinct from every role you play;

5. That you act according to role not feelings;

6. That you allow the situation to determine your role, and your role to determine behavior;

7. That service to others is the principle and purpose of all human behavior;

8. That you can't know and appreciate yourself until you do likewise to others.

CHAPTER 9

HOW TO MEDITATE

"Meditation is seeing food as it really is."

Meditation is a *concentrated* way of becoming centered via detachment. This whole book, has been about meditation – how to become emotionally balanced by thinking, feeling and eating from a conscious distance instead of emotional attachment. The centered mind is the panacean remedy for virtually every human condition – including the control of one's appetite or eating disorder. Centeredness *is* the correction factor, *is* the central organizing principle of self-control. That's what meditation is and what it's for. The only difference here is that here you'll "practice" detachment in a *concentrated* setting instead of during moment to moment daily activity.

A concentrated practice provides the extra power necessary to overcome the inertia of a well-established wrong-eating habit. Business as usual doesn't take any effort, but change requires an exertion of energy. It's easy to push a car once you get it rolling, but when it's stopped, it takes a lot more effort. Meditation empowers you by unstopping you. It makes you unstoppable.

The Detachment Meditation Exercise

Paul Gauguin said, "I shut my eyes in order to see." Meditation is the relaxation of the mind through observing its activity from a distance. You can't relax the mind using willpower – as you may have noticed, but when you simply witness it from a distance – it relaxes by itself. The problem, especially for beginners, is that we tend to be easily distracted – likewise when we're eating. It's difficult to be calmly centered for more than a few seconds without being carried away or lost in our thoughts, feelings or moment to moment activities – which is the definition of being "out of control." During meditation, you'll practice "self-remembrance" by noticing when the mind has wandered as soon as you can, then returning to controlled attention again and again. With practice, distractions occur less and less frequently and last for shorter periods of time.

To help keep you from being too easily distracted, you may want some object upon which to fix your attention while meditating, something that will serve as an *anchor* to help prevent attention from wandering. There are many devices for this purpose depending on how new you are at this, or how mentally active a personality you are – a high-strung Type A, or an easy-going Type B, for instance.

The object we'll use here is *breath-counting,* but it can be staring gently at a lighted candle, a spot on the wall, a flower, or a picture of a beloved or special person. It could be repeating some mantra, affirmation, syllable or name, or concentrating on an imaginary symbol or on the movement of one's naval, and so on; again, depending on your experience, cultural background, personality or state of mind. We'll use a breath-counting meditation because it's a natural and powerful one; one that's been practiced and proven over thousands of years by all the major religions and philosophies, and one that's compatible with the busy lifestyle of the computer-age, multi-tasking westerner.

Formal sitting meditation practice consists of four main elements: focus attention between your eyebrows; count your out-breaths; notice when anything distracts you; then return attention to breath-counting again and again. That's all there is to it. Let's look at the details.

It is suggested that formal meditation be practiced at least twice-daily, first thing in the morning, then in the early evening or at bedtime. Preferably at a regular time and place, and for periods of about 20- to 30-minutes per session. It's better to meditate before eating than after. A full stomach decreases sensitivity because the digestive process uses so much energy. Emerge from the session gently, ideally using some kind of pleasant timer. A timer prevents you from having to think about how long you've been meditating – an unnecessary distraction.

Attitude

The right attitude is important to success in meditation. The right attitude means that meditation shouldn't be regarded casually but considered as valuable and necessary to well-being as proper exercise, nutrition, and sleep. Or rather, it should be considered more important than these things, for unless you're in the right frame of mind, you won't be relaxed, motivated to exercise, eat properly, sleep or function very well. The quality of every area of your life depends on the grounded tranquility of your mind; therefore, make the twice-daily practice of meditation a top priority. Let it be the foundation of your day, the center around which all other activities revolve.

Preparation

Sit in a comfortable chair with your back and neck relatively straight. This facilitates breathing and the flow of energy and intelligence which must travel the spine to the brain. Feet should be flat and hands should be touching in some way to help concentrate energy and prevent its escaping. You may also meditate lying down, but be careful of falling asleep – unless that's what you want to do. Put aside all family, business, and personal concerns. There's a time for everything, and this is the time for the luxury and necessity of total freedom, peace and solitude.

Relaxing the Body

Begin by closing your eyes softly the way a baby does. You don't want to strain them. Then close your mouth gently and breathe normally through your nose. Then scan your body to locate and relax any physical tension. Whatever muscle you detachedly focus attention on will relax. There are many methods to relax the body. We'll use a progressive tension/release method that takes several minutes. With practice you'll be able to do it faster. You'll contract each muscle group, in order, for about five seconds each, then relax them.

First, tighten and furrow the forehead and eyebrows for a count of five – then relax them. Scrunch up your eyes and hold them tense for five seconds – then relax them. Let all the tiny muscles and nerves around the eyes relax. Scrunch up your face for five seconds, then release the tension. Be aware of the skin and muscles of your face settling, smoothing out. Allow the jaw to slightly sag. Tighten up your shoulders for five seconds – then let them slacken. Tighten up your forearms; hold – then release. Curl your fingers into tight fists – hold, then loosen them. Tighten up your chest, hold – then relax. Tighten up your buttocks and abdominal muscles, hold – then relax them. Tighten your thighs – then relax them. Tighten the calves of your legs – then relax them. Tense up all the muscles of the feet and toes – then relax them. Your legs feel comfortably heavy. Finally, scan the entire body quickly to notice and relax any last traces of tension. All the muscles of your body should now feel loose, limp and relaxed.

Focusing between Eyebrows

Now that your body is relaxed, softly focus attention to a point slightly upwards between the eyebrows and hold it there. This is the pineal gland area of the brain, sometimes called the "third eye," where thoughts surfacing from the subconscious first dawn into awareness. When we're straining to remember something, we instinctively look up toward this area. By fixing attention there, like a cat at a mouse-hole, you can catch and observe thoughts at the very point of their arising. This "being present at the inception of thought" is the heart and essence of meditation practice. This is being centered, poised, relaxed and receptive; and is the state you want to carry with you, to the degree possible, throughout the day – especially while eating. Remember that it's virtually impossible to overeat when your mind is centered.

While eating, you're "watching attentively for the hunger to subside, " here, you're watching attentively for distracting thoughts to arise. It's the same idea. Thought control, emotion control, and appetite control are all one and the same activity. To the degree you get a distance from them, they *must* submit to your wishes.

Begin by just *listening* for a few minutes. Sound itself is a powerful meditation object. Listen to any and all sounds coming from all around you. Maybe you can hear passing traffic. A bird is singing. People talking in the distance. The falling rain. Wind rustling the leaves. Just listen silently. If there's no sound, just listen to the silence. Go on listening and listening, and soon the mind becomes quieter and quieter. Soon the mind becomes totally silent and still.

Follow Your Breathing

Now while attention is focused softly between your eyes – or on the back of your eyelids, if that's more comfortable, be *very* aware of your breath inhaling, turning around, then exhaling; in, reversing, and out. Watch your breathing from a distance, as if you are an outside observer of your breathing. Be as if a witness to your breathing. Whether you're thinking something, feeling something, eating something or engaged in any activity whatsoever, remember this: If you're not *witnessing* that activity, it means that you're not detached and not in control; it means that you're virtually in a trance.

Detachment Meditation is doing two things at the same time: It's holding attention between your eyebrows *while* observing your breathing at the same time. You want to acutely witness your breathing while noticing any distracting thoughts and feelings – just as you witness your stomach while eating. It gets easier with practice.

You may breathe normally or even a bit deeper than normal. Just flow along with the breathing as it is. Don't go ahead of it or lag behind it; just be simultaneous with it, in unison with it. Join it as it moves in, curls around, and moves out; in, around, and out. Try especially to notice the very subtle gaps or transition points between the in-breath and the out-breath. Meditation is the *space* between your breaths, the space between your thoughts.

(At this point you may continue on to count your breaths or you may begin repeating affirmations or mantras as described in Chapter 1.)

Counting Your Breaths

Now start counting your out-breaths from one to ten, then repeat that ten-count for the rest of the session. Counting works as a mantra to help still the mind. *Mantra* is a Hindu word that means instrument of thought. After you've had some experience with formal meditation practice, you may not need to count any longer – again, depending on whether you're a type A or type B, etc. On the out-breath, say "one" either to yourself or quietly out loud. Continue to ten, then repeat – while at the same time, watching your breathing *as if* through your "third eye."

Noticing Distractions

Whenever you notice your mind has wandered, gently return objective attention to your breathing again and again. If you lose count, just start over without thinking anything of it. Each time a random thought breaks your silence, notice it has, then return to being detachedly aware of your breathing again and again. Don't be annoyed or impatient with yourself for taking so long to notice these distractions. With practice, you'll become more and more alert and responsive. Intruding thoughts or feelings are not the problem; getting carried away with them is.

Remember, meditation has no goal or object, per se. You cannot win at it or lose at it; it's an end in and of itself. There are great benefits, but we don't do it for the benefits; we do it because that's how being conscious works. That's how to *be* conscious. Meditation is just being objectively, impersonally, and choicelessly aware, in and of the present moment, regardless of content.

Here is a powerful device to help increase awareness during both the formal meditation and during normal daily activity: Imagine that your breathing is *not* an automatic process, and that you *have to remember to breathe*; and that if you forget to breathe or get distracted from it for too long, you'd suffocate just as if you were underwater for too long.

Meditation isn't hypnosis; it's just the opposite. Meditation is the antidote to hypnosis. It frees you from the past and present hypnotic influences of the world. You're in a "trance" right now in the sense that you're under the sway of past conditioning, training, environment, memories, beliefs and emotions — including that eating-for-comfort habit. You're hypnotized in that you're unwittingly susceptible to outside influences instead of your own inner influences.

The hypnotized person doesn't know he's in a trance. He thinks he's himself. My friend, Maxie Pierpont was put in a trance by a stage hypnotist and told to walk around in his underwear. As Maxie returned to his seat without his pants on, the audience roared with laughter. Maxie didn't know why they were laughing. He had no idea he was still "under." He knew he had no pants on but *didn't think anything of it.* It was not until the hypnotist snapped his fingers to break the trance that Maxie realized the truth.

We're all walking around in our underwear in the sense that we're being manipulated either by the past, or by someone else's idea of what we should be, do, buy or believe. As the hypnotist snapped his fingers to return Maxie to reality, so meditation works to snap us back to our real, original, un-programmed self.

Meditation itself is not mental concentration either. Mental concentration implies effort or force of will, which is energy-draining. In meditation, we are alert, paying focused attention, but there isn't any exertion involved. We're merely focusing attention in a particular direction rather than having it inefficiently scattered. This will, of course, take some getting used to, and this is where effort is required. Meditation, consciousness, life itself, is effortless; it's getting there that takes some effort and discipline.

Discipline

Meditation is more accurately a *discipline* than a concentration exercise. Learning to meditate, like learning anything new, will take patience and perseverance, but no other endeavor will bring such immeasurable rewards − especially the reward of natural appetite control.

Meditation is two things as the same time: It's both the centered state to which you aspire, and the technique to get you there. The technique itself can be learned in a few minutes, but the meditative state is what has to be discovered on your own through disciplined practice. This may take a few days, weeks, months, even years. The experience itself is simply a feeling of heightened awareness and deep tranquillity, although you may sometimes experience rapturous levels of peace and joy. But be careful to not be seduced by the egotistical promise and temptation of pleasure. Remember that you're not doing it to "get high" or get "enlightened"; you're doing it to *be* your higher self. The wrong motivation here, as we discussed in Chapter 1, will give you the opposite of what you want, will sabotage your efforts. You have to maintain an impersonal, dispassionate attitude at all times no matter the effects or results.

The simple, detached "watching" of thoughts and feelings, in and of itself, *is* to control them. Again, you can't stop mental chatter by willpower, but when you just witness it from a distance – it stops. It relaxes. You've effectively gotten above thoughts and feelings, and are no longer personally identified with them. They are no longer who or what you are. You are only a witness and nothing else. If you're not witnessing, you're identifying. You think it's you when it's really not.

Resentment, for instance, is seen as not you, but as a merely powerless thing that's happening below you by a lower faculty. Notice thoughts running like characters on a movie screen or like clouds in the sky just drifting past you. Get that you are not your thoughts or feelings but are the choiceless, impersonal witness that is above them all.

To meditate is to become aware of the mind's mechanism, memory, thoughts, desires, fantasies. The traffic is almost always there like a big city intersection at rush-hour. You have to just stand on the sidewalk and watch whatever is passing, without commentary or criticism. Just be a silent mirror reflecting whatever's passing by. Remain above the fray.

You're not concerned with *what* the mind thinks or *what* the heart feels; that's irrelevant and not the business of neutral awareness. Your only concern is to closely watch it whatever and whenever it thinks or feels. The idea is to be perfectly still in order to discern the slightest movement as an animal does when it senses something amiss. You stand merely as a *reference point* from which you're able to discern all things with greatest clarity. Notice when thoughts or feelings arise, then let them go at the same time. Dissolve them. Hold your awareness in advance of thought or feeling. Anticipate their coming. Be ready for them. And when they come, just let them evaporate in the great energy of your detached awareness – like the sun evaporates the fog.

You don't want to be blank or closed; that's not the idea. The idea is to stay openly and choicelessly aware of anything that distracts you from your silent breathing. If you feel an itch, just scratch it. If you hear a bird call, or smell food cooking, think nothing of it. When a random thought arises – and it will, just notice it has then drop it as simultaneously as possible.

The same with feelings – of perhaps boredom, impatience, restlessness, irritation, etc., witness and drop them at once. The same when you feel an inordinate craving for food – just notice it and drop it at the same time. Don't judge it or indulge it. Just drop it. Change the subject. Move on to the next creative moment. Come from your creative source not from the powerlessness of your subconscious habit.

Meditation lets you see first hand that you can think or feel without stress and without having to act on anything you don't want to act on. Just return detached

attention to your breathing again and again. Meditation puts the body, mind and spirit back into their balanced and proper relationship; that is, with the spirit (detached consciousness) leading and the body/mind following, and all working together as a single, powerful, harmonious unit.

Mental Activity

During meditation you'll experience three general types of mental activity. The first and most common type is *day dreaming.* Day dreaming is when the mind is not directed and just wanders off on its own stream of consciousness. One thought reminds you of another, which triggers another, and so on. It's idle reverie, fantasy, nostalgia; it's the musing of a hope or a wish being fulfilled; it's reliving the events of last night or last year, etc. This is not meditation, so as often as you catch yourself doing it, return objective awareness to your breathing. This is how to eat as well. If you're not eating in this "meditative" way, then you're eating in the powerlessness of your subconscious program.

We can refer to the second type of mental activity as *contemplation,* which is another word for deliberative or conscious thinking. Contemplation is the weighing or studying of an issue. It's creative brainstorming or attempting to solve some personal or business problem, etc. Contemplation is of a higher class of thought than daydreaming because it's more directed and productive, and is done more consciously; but it's in a lower class than insight or intuitive knowing which is *knowledge without thinking at all.* So whenever you find yourself contemplating instead of meditating, patiently return attention to your breathing again and again.

Insight is the third result of regular meditation practice. Insight is not mental activity as in the above cases. In fact, it's no activity at all: Insight is an experience of *direct and immediate knowing* without the intervention of thought. It emanates from the infinite storehouse of subconscious intelligence. Insights are elucidating glimpses of reality; it's seeing into the true nature of some aspect of yourself or the world – especially as it relates to eating.

Insights may be quite profound and frequent during the first few weeks or months of meditation – because they're new. Thereafter, they become increasingly subtle – because they are then accepted as perfectly normal. Some insights may be beautiful beyond words, and you may laugh or cry with joy. And some may be painful – as real or imagined events and fears from the past spring up from the subconscious mind to be seen clearly and completely for the first time. Here, too, you may laugh or cry with joy – the joy of relief and catharsis, for as these emotions bubble up, purge and dissipate before your eyes, so does all the tension that went with them. As a result, you'll feel cleansed, purified, light, refreshed, relaxed, changed, born again, renewed – not hungry any longer.

Meditation does for accumulated tension what dreams do for daily tension. One purpose of sleep dreaming is to relax the emotional tension built up during the day, so you'll wake refreshed mentally as well as physically. Dreams stimulate emotional release in the same way movies do: A tragic story releases tears; a comedy releases laughter. When the hero finally frees himself from his dangerous predicament, some of our own fear is relaxed as well. We identify with the hero's fear. While the drama in movies, books and dreams provides some relief of superficial tension, it's not powerful enough to break up the tension accumulated from childhood. For this we need to meditate. Meditation is both a means by which repressed tension may surface and dissolve, and a state of mind by which it can't return. Consciously or unconsciously, you are always on the path to centered relaxation; meditation just makes it consciously deliberate. It amplifies and accelerates the process, saving you years of painful and expensive trial and error.

When an experience of insight or revelation occurs, however major or minor, just experience it fully and indifferently, then return to your breathing again. In cases where, for example, some original idea occurs to you, or the solution to some problem presents itself, you may want to interrupt the meditation and write it down so as not to forget it or be distracted by it. But be careful not to use meditation as a brainstorming session – brainstorm in a separate session.

Now insight and intelligence are one and the same thing, and are the chief benefits of meditation – along with health, happiness and appetite-control; but the only way to cultivate it is to be indifferent to it. We don't want to be insightful or intelligent just for a moment here and there, or just when meditating; we want to be happy, intelligent and in control *always*. And the way to be so, is to be detached and indifferent *always*. Experience an insight to the fullest, but don't get carried away by it in the slightest. In this way, moments of insight will progressively widen from a split second in duration, to a minute, to an hour, to a day, to all the time. You want to live in a state of constantly detached awareness to the best of your ability.

Effects and Benefits

You'll emerge from most meditation sessions more relaxed and aware, and it will *seem* as though nothing greater is happening, but meditation works in subtle ways. The quality of your life will immediately improve, but you may not connect it to meditation because it'll all be perfectly natural. For instance, you'll find yourself working smarter instead of harder; your sense of humor and perspective will improve. All your relationships will improve as you'll become more open, tolerant, patient, loving and forgiving.

You'll be more discerning and discriminating as to friends, relationships, advisors, food, books, art, music, conversation, business opportunities, etc. Your appearance will improve as your eyes brighten, and the skin on your face tautens as vitality and alertness return to it. You'll tend to stand up straighter, with your shoulders back, and your chest out. You'll feel and express a heightened sense of confidence and well-being. In this state, your ECH is transcended and losing weight happens on its own.

Your general health will improve as the relaxation and detachment of meditation can help to control, reverse or prevent such stress-related symptoms as insomnia, high blood pressure, headaches, ulcers, many kinds of cancer, infertility, skin disease, heart disease (to name just a few), as well as dependence on substances such as alcohol, drugs, nicotine, caffeine, sugar, etc.

Meditation can achieve these benefits because it reverses the stress that triggers these ailments. Stress-related dis-ease begins in the mind, and if not checked, spreads to the body. It moves from the mental to the physical, becoming first an imperceptible microbe, then it grows to debilitating proportions. So disease, again, is the messenger, not the *real* problem; the real problem is stress – mistakenly taking life personally, self-centeredly, emotionally instead of detachedly. Self-centered stress is the cause; smoking, overeating, over drinking, are the effects. So to reverse a disease, we reverse the stress; and that's what *Detachment Meditation* does – returns you to your natural and original state of centered relaxation.

As it took a while for your body to become overweight, it will take a while for it to recover after you've become relaxed. That is, you may not lose weight immediately, even though your mind is relaxedly centered, because your body is still "on a roll" so to speak, and will need a little time to detox, de-fat and adapt. Someone observed, "The older you get, the more difficult it is to lose weight, because by then your body and your fat are really good friends." Be patient and persevering. Don't give up before the "miracle" happens. Just have faith that it definitely will happen. Don't doubt yourself; doubt your doubts.

Now the medical doctor is trained to deal primarily with effects, not with causes. His job is to diagnose and treat the *symptoms* of the disease, not necessarily the disease itself. Consequently, a patient's heart disease will either return after treatment, or the stress will express itself later in some other part of the body. True healing involves eliminating the *cause,* and only *you* can do that. The doctor can reduce the pain and inflammation and slow the growth; but only you can eliminate the fuel that feeds it.

The most active ingredient in a physician's intervention is his ability to bring you to relax. The doctor can give the patient a placebo, for example, and the most terrible disease can reverse. Why? Because the patient *believed* the "medicine" would work. He relaxed, and it did! Thus, the patient really healed himself. He believed he could be healed, relaxed, and was healed. Albert Schweitzer said "All healing is self-healing." The doctor's medicine, "bedside manner" or rapport, serve merely to compensate for the patient's inability to relax and detach – get out of the way and let the healing forces of nature run their course.

When you step on a nail, a pain chemical is released to inform the brain that a "false" object is sticking in your foot and to please remove it as soon as possible. At the same time, other agents come to eject the nail, disinfect the area, stop the bleeding, and begin grafting the torn skin back together. Emotional pain also indicates that something is wrong, that some foreign, false, or negative thought or act has invaded the mind. Now just as the first step in physical healing is to remove the nail, the first step in emotional healing is to remove or control the negative thought or feeling. As the nail is false to the body, so negativity and its accompanying stress is false or anathema to the mind. The nail is real in the sense that it's certainly sticking in your foot and certainly hurts, but is false in that it doesn't belong there. It isn't natural. It isn't a birthright. Likewise, negativity of any name or nature is real in that it does exist, but false in that it doesn't belong there. It's artificial. Emotional pain is a temporary and useful messenger. Letting it get under your skin, or get you down, means you're misunderstanding it or misusing it – and consequently overeating over it.

Let's look for a few minutes at "meditation" during normal daily activity.

Sensual Awareness

The idea here is to keep a little space between the sense organs and the objects they sense. It's to perceive things independent of your thoughts or feelings about them. It's to be keenly alert and responsive to what you perceive, yet consciously removed at the same time. In other words, you don't want to be caught up with, or dragged down to the level of, whatever your sensing or eating.

Be more detachedly indifferent to odors. Is the smell gross like the secretion ejected from a skunk, or is it pleasant and appealing like the aroma of fresh-baked bread? Is it pungent and pervasive like garlic or Limburger cheese, or sweet and delicate like the perfume of a flower or the bouquet of a good wine? Let the *nose* discriminate among aromas, but let the awareness regard all aromas as the same, as *just* aromas.

Be more detachedly indifferent to internal and external *physical feelings*. Is a thing warm or cold? moist or dry? soft or hard? Is it smooth like satin or gritty and grainy like sandpaper? Notice any physical pain, tension, or discomfort. Where exactly is it? and what is the quality and character of it? Is it in the shoulders, stomach, lower back or in the head? What part of the head, front, back, or side? How far forward or back? How small or large an area does it take up? Is it a dull pain, or a sharp, piercing, biting or throbbing pain? The mental energy you direct toward pain, whether physical or emotional, is the same energy that relaxes that pain. To pay very close, detached attention to your physical discomfort is all that's necessary to controlling or reversing it — just as you earlier relaxed your muscles by simply focusing on them. It's impossible for pain and awareness to exist in the same place at the same time. The only problem, of course, is that we're not aware, not *objectively* aware.

Be more detachedly indifferent to how a food *tastes*. Is it sweet like honey and strawberries, or sour, tart and tangy like lemon or vinegar? Is it salty like ham and pork, or bland like bean curd? Is it bitter, briny, minty, metallic, rancid, nutty, peppery, acrid, spicy, zesty? Let the flavors begin in your mouth and end in your mouth. Don't let them travel to the emotions to be abused or distorted. Let the *tongue* discriminate among tastes, but let the awareness regard all tastes as equal. The key to increased awareness is for each organ or faculty to know its proper place and to not co-mingle: It's for the tongue to taste, the heart to feel, the mental to think, and the consciousness to remain above it all. That's appetite control!

Be more detachedly indifferent to *sound*. What do you hear, and what is the quality and character of that sound? Is it a clang, a bellow, a blare, a rattle, rustle, screech, chatter, crash, hiss, hum, murmur, pop, splash, squeak, sputter, fizzle, swish, tinkle? Is it loud and piercing like a siren, or soft and gentle like the purring of a kitten? Is it clear and distinct, or muted, faint, subdued, distant? Is it resonant or dissonant, full or hollow, boisterous or mellow? Is the rhythm monotonous like a whine or melodious like a song? Is it a high frequency sound like that of a flute or a whistle, or a low frequency one like that of a tuba? Is it harsh and jarring like a fingernail scraping against a chalkboard, or is it soothing and harmonious like a passage from a Brahm's lullaby? Let sounds originate in your ear and end in your ear. Don't allow them to travel to the thinking or feelings to be contaminated. Let the ear discriminate among sounds, but let the awareness regard all sound as the same, as *just* sound.

Notice people – including yourself, with discrimination but without comment or judgment; look at their sizes, shapes, postures, movements, gestures, and facial expressions. Look at what they say and how they say it, what they do and how they do it. Notice that everyone's doing the best they can in that moment – so patience and forgiveness become so much easier.

Be more detachedly indifferent to what you *see*. Notice how light or dark things are, how transparent or opaque, pale or vivid, symmetrical or asymmetrical. Look at how blue the sky is, how low or high the clouds hang. Look at how tall, craggy, and colorful the mountains, how deep the valleys, how wide the canyons. Witness the shape and greenness of the leaves on a tree, and the texture and brownness of the bark. Notice how thick the fog and haze, how tumultuous the storm, and how the raindrops splash on the pavement. See how placid the lake, how tremendous the ocean, how swift and powerful the river, how clear and bubbly the brook, how delicate the mist on a flower.

When the senses are detached from the intellect and the emotions, things are perceived more clearly and vividly. It's like a veil or filter has been removed and you are seeing life (and food) as if for the first time. Before, everything was taken for granted, now, all things become interesting, relevant and meaningful. Things are seen to have a life, personality, and consciousness of their own. They are all communicating with each other on some level – and communicating with us as well. The language is subtle; to hear it will require a mind that is open, receptive, detached and still. Reality is as shy as a bird and the slightest movement will frighten her away. But through perfect unobtrusiveness, she'll feel related to you. She'll sit on your shoulder and reveal herself to you. A person so alive and detachedly conscious is also so naturally controlled.

Physical Awareness

Breaking the attachment or identification with the body is likewise achieved by viewing it from a distance. You want to observe the body's parts, shapes, postures, actions and reactions as if from the position of an outside observer. As you go about your business, try to catch yourself in the *middle* of some position or activity. Notice what you are doing without giving yourself any warning, as if taking a candid photograph of yourself. For example, as you are reading these words, quickly glance over at your right hand and regard it as not belonging to you. Just stop and look at it for a minute without moving it and without your mind entering into it. Notice the position of the thumb and fingers, notice the color of the skin, its texture, lines, and pores. Look at the knuckles, veins, hair and nails. Do the same when you find yourself lying down, sitting, standing, walking, etc. Sneak up on yourself and notice your posture or facial expression prior to making any self-conscious adjustments to them.

Finding, discovering, knowing yourself simply means *remembering* yourself, remembering that you are indeed above, separate, and in control of yourself. And once you regain dominion over yourself, you simultaneously regain dominion over the world and over food as well, for the two are not separate. Harmony within translates to harmony without. As you make sense, so does the world; as you fall into order, so does the world; as you become beautiful, so does the world. Detached awareness is simply the means by which to both trigger or stimulate this recollection, and to maintain it as well.

The theory behind this reality-based strategy of detachment is that in order to become natural, we must first become aware of our *un*naturalness; before we can know the truth of ourselves we must first become aware of our falseness; before we can know pleasure, we must first go through the pain; and in the same way, in order to become spontaneously *un*self-conscious, we must first be deliberately *self*-conscious. It's necessary to pass through the night in order to reach the day, to pass through the negative to reach the positive. The negative is the bridge to freedom. We begin with the negative because that's the condition we happen to be in. That's the condition we, through inheritance, happened to be born in. We detach from the negative to reach the positive, appetite-controlled state.

In all activity, be conscious of *what* you're doing and *how* you're doing it. Again, these are the only two questions awareness is concerned with. Awareness is not concerned with *why* you are doing a particular thing. "Why" is a function of the lower mental faculty. "Why" is an academic concept, but awareness is experiential. Life is not to be thought about and questioned in this context; it's to be known and lived. Thinking and questioning miss the point. Life is to be known directly, immediately, wholly, and completely. Remember, you want to live and eat in such a way as to be above and independent of the lower faculties. You want to experience life and food in and of themselves, without attachment to them. And the way you accomplish this is by being detachedly attentive to *what* you're doing and *how* you're doing it. Nothing else. What kind of work do you do and how do you do it? If you are a manager, what are you managing and how are you managing it? If you are a trial attorney, what is the evidence you are presenting and how are you presenting it? If you are a surgeon, what procedure are you performing and how are you performing it? If working on an assembly line, what are you assembling and how? When smoking cigarettes, notice how you hold the cigarette and how you flick the ashes. Notice the smoke being inhaled and exhaled. How does it smell? How does it taste and feel in your mouth and on your throat? Do this with every drag and you'll soon stop smoking because consciousness is now overruling the subconscious – where the habit is embedded.

What leisure activities are you involved in and how? In listening to music or viewing a work of art, notice how compatible it is with your highest sense of harmony, and witness what feelings they evoke. When reading or watching a drama, be aware of what the main character wants, what's preventing him from getting it, how he goes about achieving it, how he succeeds or fails, and what is the theme or moral of the story. Be conscious that your own life has these same dramatic elements. What do you want? What's hindering you? How are you going about attaining it? What obstacles are you struggling to overcome? What lessons must you learn? And what's the theme, meaning or purpose of your own life? And the same applies to your subconscious eating habit: To the degree you objectively notice what and how you're eating – the unwanted habit lets *you* go!

The meditative state and the objective state are one and the same state of mind. We refer to them by different names depending on when "practiced." During daily activity, it's being centered; when in a formal, structured setting, it's called meditation. We want to experience life and food as a present-moment fact, not as a figment of the imagination. We want to experience life and food in its innocence and nakedness, not clothed in the projections of our fantasies and emotional expectations.

Key Points and Principles to Remember from this Chapter:

1. – That formal meditation is the concentrated practice of being centered via detached awareness of all that you see, hear, think, feel and do;

2. – That meditation practice consists of relaxing the body, focusing attention between the eyebrows, counting out-breaths from 1-10, witnessing distractions without comment, and returning attention to breath-counting again and again;

3. – That meditation practice enhances physical, sensual, mental and emotional awareness;

4. – That meditation practice relaxes physical, mental and emotional stress;

5. – That affirmations should be simple, positive, in the present tense, and stated with an attitude of gratitude, humility and the assumption that they will be fulfilled.

CHAPTER 10

HOW TO BE PRESENT

"The past is a guidepost, not a hitching post."

– L. Thomas Holdcroft

Neither the past nor the future are "real," so neither has the power to control your mind or body. The present moment is the point of the six C's: calmness, contentment, centeredness, clarity, control and confidence. Only here and now can the mind be relaxed, satisfied and objectively aware. Being present means total involvement in, and knowledge of, what you're thinking, feeling and eating. It means your attention isn't divided or conflicted.

When eating, showering, dressing or driving, for instance, notice that your mind is only partially there. And if you trace your activities through the day, you'll see that the mind is seldom on the thing at hand – especially eating. This, not living or eating in the present, is equal to the uncentered, uncontrolled, overweight state of mind.

We think we're more productive when "multi-tasking," for example, but the reverse is true: Not focusing on one thing at a time, in the present, makes us less productive and intelligent because the energy of awareness is dissipated and diffused.

We're scatterbrained. We don't know what a shower feels like. We don't know what food tastes like. We don't remember a peoples' names, what we just read, etc. We're like a person in a day-dream or trance who misses his exit on the highway, or like a drunk in a blackout who makes it home, but doesn't have a clue how he did it. The idea that the mundane is not worthy of awareness is to miss the point that the present is the point of clarity and appetite-control power regardless of the object.

If you're not present in the shower, you won't be very present in other situations either – like while eating, for example – because you're out of practice. Your awareness has become lethargic or atrophied. Being present is not only a discipline, it's the mother of all disciplines, for if you're not all here, you're not all there. The saying "Use it or lose it" applies to the higher faculty of consciousness as it does to thinking, feeling, and the five senses. In fact, it applies especially to the higher, for the higher consciousness is your *central guidance or reference point* by which you can control all the lower faculties.

Remember that any mind/body transformation can only occur in the present moment: Only in the present can you be detachedly conscious, maintain your new self-image, control your appetite and portions, exercise your body, and manage your stress.

Overcoming Temptation

To be effective and secure, one doesn't have to refer to the past or look to the future, for both are inherent in the present and stored in your subconscious mind. The present is a self-contained universe that doesn't require anything external to it. Anything from the past that would be useful and relevant to this moment will spontaneously spring up from the subconscious and be available to you. It's always at hand. You don't have to "remember" that all actions have consequences; you just have to be alert in the present moment. When so alert, all ramifications and resolutions present themselves simultaneously. Before you eat beyond satiety, for example, you won't have to "think it through," for you'll know very well the ramifications of such a mindless act because – via present-moment detachment, you are no longer mindless.

Temptation is no longer a factor. You transcend it. It's a low and obsolete emotion that you've gone beyond. Yes, you'll still feel temptation on occasion because it's been part of your mindset your whole life. It's part of the human condition. The point is now you don't have to *act* on it. You have a choice now. Just because you *feel* like eating the wrong food at the wrong time, doesn't mean you have to *act* on it. It's okay to *think* of shooting someone, but you don't actually do it. Momentary discomfort is not the end of world. It always passes, and you feel so much better about yourself for not succumbing. Success builds on success. Confidence builds on confidence.

Present-moment detachment increases your emotional intelligence. If you're in the past – *remembering* the "comfort" you got from food, or if you're in the future – *anticipating* the "comfort" that a gratuitous extra helping might bring you – then you'll succumb. In the present moment, right and wrong present themselves simultaneously, so that the choice becomes clear. The way to go becomes obvious. It's not complicated; it's just about doing what you know is right, and if you're present, you'll have the power to do so.

The Present is the Point of Security

If a person is alert in the present, the future will provide for itself; if not, nothing from the past will help. By living from the past, he'll either repeat the same mistakes over and over, or make different ones all the time. He'll find himself always "chalking things up to experience," doing and saying the wrong thing at the wrong time, not being quite "with it." Always being "a day late and a dollar short." Reality is happening, but he'll be constantly out of sync with it, constantly lagging a bit behind because he must always refer to his memory before responding. Even if it's for just a split-second, it's too late. The moment has passed. The boat has been missed. He overeats. Life is happening *now* and must be responded to *now.* To miss by only a hair is still to miss. To eat just an ounce beyond satiety will keep you overweight.

The ordinary person erroneously "believes" that by leaving his comfort zone of the past, he'd be as if lost in space, without any point of reference. He needs something to hang onto, some kind of security blanket – which in this case is food.

So the person not fully present lives in a false sense of security. False because he's no more secure than an ostrich hiding its head in the sand. Responding to life and food correctly and confidently, is based on knowing what's happening *right now,* and the only way to know, is to *be there* right now.

The experience of the past is a secondary and inferior consideration. The past is academic; the present is real life, lived in real time. It's whole and complete so is free of error, uncertainty, and the need to overeat. A rule of thumb is this: When you're anxious, you're in the future; when depressed, you're in the past. When you're not detachedly present, you're in doubt, fear and error. When present, you're living from your higher subconscious mind, the foundation of all clarity, confidence and appetite-controlling knowledge and power.

The Present is The Point of Freedom

All of our thinking and feeling happens in and out of the present; and in order for the mind to be responsive to what's happening outside of it, it must be *flexible and free.* The more free, the more adaptable to lightning-fast, moment-to-moment activity. In order for awareness to keep up, it must move at the same speed as reality, and paradoxically, the only way it can do that is to remain perfectly relaxed and responsive. Then there's no time or space for past conditioning to inveigle itself into your stomach.

The present is equal to the meditation state where your attention is focused at the intersection of consciousness in order to notice the slightest movement. Mental stillness and presence of mind are one and the same state. As soon as the mind leaves stillness to become emotional – you've left the moment as well. The rule of thumb is this: If your mind is still, you are here; if it's going, you are gone. *To maintain the present moment, just maintain your detached, witnessing mindset.* It's virtually impossible to overeat in the present moment because the inherent power of the present neutralizes any unwanted desire or habit.

The present moment and the tension-free state of centeredness are the same. The present is like neutral gear in an automobile, the position in which there's no "stress" on the engine, and the position in which the car is now poised to move in any direction at any time. The future and past are like the forward and reverse gears; they are the positions of movement or emotion. In the forward position you can't go backwards; and in reverse you can't go forward. So you're not only stressed, but limited to only one position at a time. To choose one position is to sacrifice the other. In any given moment, half your potential is denied. But in present-moment reality, you can move in neutral, forward and reverse, all at the same time.

How? Because emotional movement and creative movement work in different directions: Emotional energy moves horizontally, while creative energy moves vertically. Emotional movement is toward the future or the past; but creative movement is inward and outward. By conceiving inwardly and expressing it outwardly, you're not only able to travel in "neutral")centeredness(, and travel without stress, but you can travel in both forward and reverse at the same time as well – for as you move, you pull the entire past and the entire future along with you simultaneously. When you move in the right direction, the whole universe, all knowledge, moves with you.

You want to live and eat spontaneously, by common sense and intuition – as if you never really lived before nor tasted food before. Freedom is living in accordance with how things *really* are, not with how you *think* they are. Thinking takes time but life is constant. Thinking is living around life, not in and to life. In order to be sensitive and receptive to the ever-changing newness of it, the old must be continually dropped. We cannot write on a chalkboard filled with yesterday's scribbles; it must first be erased. Otherwise the past will not only influence, affect and interfere with the present, it will *prevent* the present as well. If you want something, you have to make a space for it.

Freedom is direct and immediate knowing and responding. It's a state of total flexibility and open-mindedness where there's no time or space between what's happening and a response that's appropriate to it. You are connected to the moment as directly and harmoniously as a dancer to his partner. When he moves forward, she simultaneously moves backwards, and vice versa. Their movements are not thought about or premeditated, and exactly *because* they are not, a perfect synchrony is automatically and effortlessly maintained. They've acquired "muscle memory" and have let go of mental memory. That's what you want to do: acquire "detachment memory" in order to maintain transcendence over your eating-for-comfort memory.

To live from the past is like suffering a permanent hangover. When we eat or drink too much, the next day is affected. Instead of waking to a new day refreshed and alert, the mind and body remain dull and heavy. We're not free to relax and enjoy today because of yesterday's residue. Yesterday is no longer real or relevant but merely a concept, a memory. To have our lives controlled and determined by the past is a denial of the present – which is a denial of reality itself. As physical hangovers are of the past so are psychological and emotional hangovers. We overeat because we think that's just the way we are. We lived in our program and didn't know it like a fish lives in water and doesn't know it.

Each moment is as unique as a fingerprint. You're not the same person you were a moment ago and if alive, won't be the same person a moment from now either. The experience of this moment will change you so that you'll act and respond in a new and different way in the next moment. This is true freedom and attachment to anything whatsoever – especially to food, is the very killer of it.

There are no good or bad experiences as far as neutral, objective awareness is concerned; there are only different and changing experiences, like clouds passing in the sky. The nature of reality is constant change and growth. Change is the only thing in life that is permanent. Heraclitus said, "You cannot step in the same river twice." To cling to the taste of past pleasures is a denial of present-moment life, growth and reality. Each moment is a different snowflake, a different miracle. Carbon copies cannot exist among that which is alive but only with things that are dead. Only the dead are the same yesterday, today and tomorrow; the living are always moving, growing, creating. The person who clings to life keeps missing it. Or, in the words of the master of detachment, "Whosoever would save his)self-centered(life will lose it."

The person who clings to the past is like a cartoon character working on an assembly line in a bottling factory. The conveyor belt is constantly moving, and if he spends too much time on the present bottle, the next one crashes to the floor, and when he tries to save it the next one falls, then the next, and the next. Or it's like a clerk in a doughnut shop who doesn't rotate the doughnuts properly: He puts the fresh ones in back and leaves the stale ones in front, so customers always get the stale ones, never the fresh ones.

Life is always fresh, but becomes stale when we live in the past or the future. We cannot cling to anything in life because it's happening too fast, and we can't escape anything either because we're surrounded by it. The only choice remaining is to let go and flow along with it. Be indifferent to it. And in that holy indifference lies the relaxation and appetite-control we had been searching for all along. When the dog finally becomes frustrated and exhausted enough from chasing his own tail, he lies down to rest, only to find his tail brushing his lips.

Living with a Passion

If at any given moment, most of your attention is directed either toward the past or toward some future event or result – like your weight loss goal, then less energy and intelligence remains to facilitate achieving that goal. If you have one eye on the future, you'll have only one eye left with which to live in the goal. Living in the goal instead of the future is to already be there. This principle applies to your moment- to-moment goals as well as to long term goals. The present is both the point of desire and the point of attainment. If you're not present you'll miss it.

The moment at hand is the entrance to life, the entrance to truth – its blood is to be drunk and its flesh is to be eaten. Our task is to enter this moment and to realize and accept that there's no end to it. When Robin Hood's opponent hit the bull's-eye, everyone "believed" the game was over and began to leave. But Robin Hood didn't believe it – and proceeded to split the arrow. This moment is like the arrow at the center of the bull's-eye – it can be split indefinitely. To the degree you remain in the center of the moment, the center of your goal, there's no end to the game; to the degree you look forward or backward, the game is over.

The idea is to experience this moment so completely that nothing of it is left over to carry and weigh you down. You want to enter the moment cleanly and leave it cleanly. You want to end the moment when the moment is ended, not leave it with unresolved questions or with hangovers of resentment, doubt, regret, guilt. Let what comes up in the moment also go down with it. Have no unfinished business. Find your house clean and leave it clean. Settle an issue on the spot. If the bully of temptation and craving isn't stood up to there and then, it will trouble you always. Make all your actions complete and total. A sharpshooter doesn't aim, *then* fire, he aims and fires simultaneously. There's no space between the aiming and the firing; it's a single, unified action. Let the moment be the same – single, unified, all-inclusive. Let it come out of itself and return to itself.

Penetrate each moment with calmness and contentment and leave it the same way; that is, without accumulating anything in the process, such as the desire that the next moment be the same or different. To the degree you remain in the present, all the knowledge necessary to overcome any eating issue will be spontaneously available to you.

You are being constantly guided by an inner)subconscious(sense or spirit of wholeness. This spirit is what tells you what course of action to take in all circumstances, what to say and not to say, what to do and when to do it, what to eat and when to stop eating, etc. This harmonizing spirit wants you and your goals to become one happy whole. In present-moment detachment you become receptive to its direction and empowered to fulfill it. You become guided from within.

Seizing the Moment

Centeredness via detachment can come by degree, or all at once. You can gradually become relaxedly centered over a period of weeks, months or years; or, in a single spontaneous let-go, decades of residual tension can relax in a flash. The instant route is, of course, more appealing, but spontaneity cannot be premeditated; it's an obvious contradiction. You'll either become spontaneously centered or you won't, but you can't plan it. What you can do, however, is stay ready and receptive so that, in the first place, it *can* come, and in the second place, when it does, you'll *be there.* The nature of spontaneity is to delight by surprise, but if you're never home, or the doors and windows of your mind are closed, you'll keep missing and missing. It's like the door-to-door salesman who needs only one sale per day to earn a living, but in order to make that one sale, he must knock on fifty doors. And just as the salesman can't know in advance which house contains the buyer, you can't know at which moment blissful centeredness will come, but must remain ready, alert, and receptive at *every* moment. Again, don't give up before the "miracle" happens, and the miracle *must* happen because that's how you were conceived; that's how the higher subconscious mind works. You just have to get out of the way – which is the whole purpose of detachment.

The present is elusive and precarious. Once you've found it, you have to hang onto it like a surfer riding the crest of a wave. The crest is his "moment." Once he's found it, he can't let it go. While riding it, he's in heaven and the very picture of grace and beauty. But if he loses it – into the sea he flops. Or it's like a rodeo cowboy riding a bucking bronco. Sitting on the bull when the bell rings and the gate swings open is the rider's moment. As long as he and the bull move as one animal, all is well; nothing negative can happen to him. But as soon as a little time or space develops between the bull's back and the cowboy's bottom – that's the end of the cowboy.

Being Already Dead

Jused as dying before one is ready is among the most tragic things, so being ready to die is among the most beautiful and slimming. And the way to be ready to die is to *assume you're dead already* – just as you're *already* at your goal weight. Accept the idea that you're already dead and that this moment is just a fluke, a miracle, an oversight on the part of existence. You're going to be dead in a few years anyway, so why not live as if today is not only the last day of your life, but the first as well? This is the same as the one-day-at-a-time approach to living and eating that we discussed in Chapter 3. Treat each day as a mini-life, as your whole life in microcosm. As if this day is all there is. Each day, from awakening to bedtime is a whole new world to enjoy and explore. Each awakening is a new birth, and each sleep is a new death. You don't fear "death" because you know it's just a rejuvenating rest period between awakenings.

The way to be free is to egotistically die to the present moment, to risk everything in it, put all your trust in it. What have you to lose but your excess mental, emotional and physical weight. Before there can be the new mind/body, the old must be let go. Before you can awaken, past programs have to be put to sleep. Life, consciousness and happiness demand that nothing be held back. Commitment has to be total and constant. There can be no looking back, no hesitation, for this moment is all there is, all there ever has been, and all there ever needs to be. Within it is realized the whole theme of existence – to relax and enjoy your beautiful mind and slimmer body.

Key Points and Principles to Remember from this Chapter:

1. – That present-moment centeredness is achieved by remaining consciously detached from the past and the future;

2. – That the present moment nullifies all past habits and conditioning;

3. – That the present moment is the point of the 6C's: Calmness, Contentment, Clarity, Control, Centeredness, and Confidence;

4. – That the present transcends emotional conflict;

5. – That the present overcomes temptation and craving;

6. – That the present is the point of comfort, security and power;

7. – That the present is the point of flexibility, spontaneity, and freedom;

8. – That depression is of the past and anxiety is of the future.

9. – That being present is about maintaining a detached, witnessing, passive mindset.

10. – That the present is the central guidance and reference point of clarity and appetite-control power.

APPENDIX

Break Your Love Affair with Food

BOOK SYNOPSIS

THE PROBLEM AND THE REMEDY

1. You've acquired the habit of eating for emotional comfort and security instead of physical nourishment;

2. This wrong purpose and relationship prevents you from controlling your appetite;

3. Detaching from this habit will regain control of your appetite;

4. You detach from this habit by thinking, feeling, and eating from a conscious *distance* instead of emotional involvement!

5. The law is this: When the unwanted eating habit is experienced *detachedly* instead of emotionally, it stops at will!

I. HOW TO RECREATE YOUR SELF-IMAGE

A. *Picture* yourself at your goal weight or size;

B. Hold the attitude that you're *already* there;

C. Feel the joy, contentedness and freedom *now* that you will feel then!

II. HOW TO CONTROL YOUR APPETITE

A. Eat slowly and detachedly, while

B. Watching very attentively for the hunger to subside,

C. Then, stop eating immediately!

III. HOW TO CONTROL YOUR PORTIONS

A. *Pre-plan* 4 meals a day w/nothing in between;

B. Weigh or measure all meals;

C. *Record* all meals to maintain due diligence.

IV. HOW TO EXERCISE YOUR BODY

A. Physical and Recreational Activities;

B. Flexibility and Strength Exercises;

C. Aerobic Activities.

V. HOW THE UNIVERSE WORKS

A. Balance is the central organizing and controlling principle of everything in the universe.

B. Balance is meant for the individual because that's how the universe works as a whole.

C. Emotional Balance nullifies all negative feelings and habits.

VI. HOW TO BE CENTERED

A. Accept the negative and the positive with equanimity;

B. Remain above all thought, feeling, desire and action;

C. Remain undisturbed by pain, unexcited by pleasure.

VII. HOW TO CONTROL YOUR STRESS

A. Keep a conscious and respectable *distance* from all you see, hear, think, feel and do;

B. Take nothing personal;

C. *Meditate* daily to cultivate and maintain detachment.

VIII. HOW TO ACT

A. Act according to role, not thought or feeling;

B. Let the situation determine your role, and the role determine your behavior;

C. Service to others is the principle and purpose of successful human behavior and relationship.

IX. HOW TO MEDITATE

A. Scan body to relax all muscle groups;

B. Focusing between eyebrows, count out-breaths, 1- 10;

C. Notice distracting thoughts without comment, and return attention to breath-counting again and again.

X. HOW TO BE PRESENT

A. Remain detached from the past and the future;

B. Remain centered between the past and the future;

C. Remain consciously and constantly above all experience.

ABOUT THE AUTHOR

Bill's formal training was in electronics engineering – a field he abandoned after he accidently discovered the "law of detachment" during a certain "spiritual awakening" experience. This led him to an intense 30-year research of human potential development. He is the author of *The Relaxation Principle, Getting Centered: The Master Key to Unconditional Happiness*, and *The Zen of Sobriety: How To Stop Drinking Without Really Trying.* Bill is a single, former Bostonian, living in Naples, Florida, where he blogs on Zen-centered living.